THE LOW-FODMAP DIET COOKBOOK FOR BEGINNERS

A Scientifically Proven Solution with over 100 Easy and Delicious Recipes for IBS Relief, Managing Digestive Disorders, and 7-Day Helpful Meal Plan

Dominique Santini

Table of Contents

Introduction

The FODMAP diet is both scientifically proven and internationally accepted as a method of controlling the symptoms of IBS and other digestive disorders. The common symptoms of IBS include nausea, pain, bloating, flatulence, vomiting and changes in bowel habits. However, what goes on in the gut has an overwhelming effect on the rest of the body and people with IBS symptoms also sometimes suffer from unexpected symptoms such as fatigue, depression and poor concentration, just to name a few.

Foods are meant to serve us, our taste, hunger, and to energize us. It becomes an anathema when what is supposed to treat it us a better experience now serves as our most prominent enemy. If what you eat makes you feel uncomfortable, then the food had not carried out its intended function. There are certain health challenges that we face. The foods we eat ought to give us the energy that we need to do whatever possible we need to do to fight the issues. However, there is an opposite case that is presently common. Foods now serve as a common trigger that helps the health issues in some people to become stronger. Rather than fight the scourge, food helps the scourge to manifest from time to time, hence the term – food intolerance.

If you're looking for a way to start your low FODMAP journey or have been on it for quite some time and are just exploring for more recipes, then this book will be your best friend.

Chapter 1: How does the low-fodmap diet work?

A low FODMAP diet, also called FODMAP elimination diet, is an eating pattern that eliminates or significantly reduces the amount of short-chain carbs and sugar alcohols, otherwise known as FODMAPs. The principle behind this diet is to allow the gut some time to heal by cutting out certain food. This is particularly helpful for people who have gastrointestinal problems like IBS and IBD.

The food that are excluded from a low FODMAP diet aren't necessarily unhealthy. Some of them contain galacto-oligosaccharides (GOS), inulin, and fructans, which are beneficial prebiotics that support the growth of good bacteria in the gut. Many of them are in fact healthy, but in some people, consuming them leads to gastrointestinal symptoms.

What are FODMAPs?

FODMAPs are types of carbohydrates that have been proven to cause digestive problems such as pain, bloating, and gas. A wide range of food products contain these harmful carbohydrates. The best way to protect yourself from the negative impact that they have on your health is to avoid consuming food products with FODMAPs in them.

Some foods contain only one type of FODMAP, while others contain several. The acronym FODMAP stands for:

Fermentable – Fermentation is a process in which bacteria break down or ferment undigested carbohydrates in the large bowel

Oligosaccharides – "saccharide" pertains to "sugar" and "oligo" indicates "few"; these molecules are comprised of individual sugars that are merged in a chain; they are commonly found in wheat, legumes, rye, some fruits and vegetables including onions and garlic; fructans and galacto-oligosaccharides are the main carb

Disaccharides – "di" means "double" or "two"; these double-sugar molecules can be found in milk, soft cheese, and yogurt; lactose is the primary carb

Monosaccharides – "mono" indicates "one" or "single"; single-sugar molecules are present in various fruits including mangoes and figs, and sweeteners like agave nectar and honey; fructose is the primary carb

Polyols – or "sugar alcohols" are found in certain vegetables and fruits including lychees and blackberries, and in chewing gums and artificial sweeteners

The most common FODMAPs in foods are:

Lactose: a type of sugar found in milk and other dairy foods

Fructose: a type of sugar found in many fruits and veggies

Fructans: quite similar to fructose; present in many grains and vegetables

Galactans: found mainly in legumes

If you eat a lot of high FODMAP food, you may experience signs and symptoms like gas, bloating, abdominal pain, abdominal distention, and diarrhea. But how exactly do FODMAPs cause these discomforts?

If poorly digested, saccharides and polyols go through a fermentation process in the lower part of the large intestines (bowel). This process pulls water in and produces hydrogen, methane gas, and/or carbon dioxide, causing the intestines to expand and stretch. This results in severe pain and other symptoms. Water being drawn into the small intestine can also cause diarrhea.

This is where the low FODMAP diet comes in. By eliminating or reducing your consumption of FODMAPs, you can improve your symptoms and manage your condition better. The Low FODMAP diet can be quite restrictive and complex. However, knowing the right food products to eat as well as a few cooking and dieting hacks can help you experience the joys of eating despite being on this diet. Remember that different people have sensitivities to different FODMAPs, so it is important to pinpoint which ones are triggering the symptoms.

Benefits of a Low FODMAP Diet There are more than 30 research studies that support the benefits of following a low FODMAP diet, as conducted among thousands of IBS patients. The logic here is simple: the diet immensely helps in reducing your digestive symptoms while improving your quality of life at the same time.

Reduces digestive symptoms Symptoms of digestive disorders such as IBS and IBD vary widely. It may include bloating, stomach pain, flatulence, reflux, and even rectal bleeding. Stomach pain is the main feature of a digestive condition, while bloating affects more than 80% of IBS patients.

Luckily, a low FODMAP diet has been shown to significantly reduce the instances of these symptoms. According to studies, following the diet can increase your chances of improving bloating and stomach pain by 75% and 81%, respectively. Many other studies also suggest that the diet can aid in managing diarrhea, constipation, flatulence, and other similar symptoms.

Improves quality of life Symptoms of a digestive disorder can be debilitating and lead to poor quality of life. In fact, a major study found that people with IBS would be willing to give up 25% (on average) of their lifespan just to be free of the symptoms. Due to severe pain, as well as to the stigma associated with the condition, social life of IBS and IBD patients also suffer.

But, by reducing symptoms through a low FODMAP diet, people with IBS and IBD can improve their quality of life and maintain healthy relationships with other members of the society. Some evidence also shows that following the diet can increase levels of energy among IBS sufferers. However, placebo-controlled research may be needed to back this finding.

Should You Follow a Low FODMAP Diet?

If you have a GI problem, you may and you should, otherwise you better not.

A low FODMAP diet is primarily used to alleviate digestion-related symptoms, particularly those of Irritable Bowel Syndrome (IBS) and Inflammatory Bowel Disease (IBD), but it is also becoming a useful treatment for other conditions, such as:

Small Intestinal Bacterial Overgrowth (SIBO)

Other types of Functional Gastrointestinal Disorder (FGID)

Some types of autoimmune diseases/conditions including multiple sclerosis, rheumatoid arthritis, and eczema

Fibromyalgia, frequent migraines, or any other health issues that seem to be triggered by specific foods

FODMAPs encourage the growth of beneficial bacteria in the gut. So, unless you've been diagnosed with IBS or any of the conditions mentioned above, following a low FODMAP diet may cause you more harm than good. It is important to get a go signal from your doctor or dietitian before switching to this diet.

Before starting the diet, you should: Make sure you really have IBS or IBD

Self-diagnosis is a big no-no. If you are experiencing recurrent stomach pain, stool symptoms, and other persistent symptoms, you should consult a doctor first before embarking on this diet. This eating pattern must also be followed under the guidance of a qualified dietitian.

Make necessary preparations Since the diet restricts a lot of food types, it can be hard to follow if you aren't well prepared. Here are a few tips:

Create a shopping list: Make a list of the low FODMAP food you need before heading to the supermarket or grocery store, so you won't need to do any guesswork. Also, make sure to carefully read the labels and list of ingredients to make sure that the products you're buying don't contain high FODMAPs.

Read menus ahead of time: Familiarizing yourself with low FODMAP menu options is particularly useful when eating out at restaurants or takeaway shops.

Additionally, it's important to note that the low FODMAP diet is a resource-and time-intensive process. As such, trying it for the first time during a stressful or busy period or while travelling may not be a good idea.

When you can start the LOW diet FODMAP?

The LOW-FODMAP diet is right for you if:

You have excess intestinal gas problems, bloating, abdominal pain, diarrhea or constipation;

You are not able to alleviate these symptoms by changing your style of food and non-food life (drinking more fluids, doing exercise, eating foods with an increased amount of dietary fiber, stress management, sleep better);

Together with your doctor you have eliminated any possible causes of irritable bowel syndrome that might be the cause of your symptoms and if your doctor has advised you to follow FODMAP method to eliminate the symptoms caused by irritable bowel syndrome.

The effectiveness of the LOW diet FODMAP

By learning to know the characteristics of FODMAP, the foods in which they are contained in excessive amounts, how to avoid them and how to gradually reintegrate into our power, we will begin to have a greater understanding of our problems and their causes. Thanks to this method, we will have a resolution of symptoms and improvement in gastrointestinal health. Generally, study the therapeutic efficacy of a diet is not very simple, both for the complexity that many diets often impose on rigid diets that are difficult to follow scrupulously; both because they require substantial changes to the lifestyle of the participants.

One potential problem in LOW-FODMAP diets is the lack of accurate data on the content of these substances in different foods. In addition, there is a difficulty in establishing the of each food consumption threshold values as it is not the content of a single food but the total FODMAP content consumed in the meal to determine the appearance or not of the symptoms.

Before you start a job like this, it would be good to talk with your doctor and possibly run the breath test at least for fructose, lactose and sorbitol to evaluate a possible malabsorption of these sugars.

The LOW-FODMAP diet is not the treatment of Irritable Bowel Syndrome: it is a diet whose aim is to reduce symptoms associated with certain pathologies. The use of diet indicated by the LOW-FODMAP has shown good efficacy and excellent results. Over 70% of the subjects that followed showed great improvements and, after the step of reintroduction of FODMAP, often allows to raise the threshold of tolerance towards trigger foods.

The Three Phases

In a low FODMAP diet, you don't actually need to eliminate all FODMAPs long-term. In fact, you should not eliminate all of them permanently because FODMAPs are instrumental for maintaining gut health.

There are three phases you need to go through in order to identify which specific carbs trigger your digestive symptoms and to modify your diet according to your personal tolerance. The three phases are equally important to achieve long-lasting relief from digestive symptoms and improved overall wellbeing. Then again, it is recommended that you undergo these steps with a qualified dietitian who will guide you through the proper foods.

Phase 1: Elimination/Restriction The first phase, known as the elimination or restriction phase, lasts about 3 to 8 weeks, depending on how you respond. During this stage, you strictly avoid or exclude all high FODMAP foods from your diet.

Some people experience improvement in their digestive symptoms in as early as the first or second week, while others can take the full 8 weeks. Once you've felt enough relief from your symptoms, you can move on to the second phase.

The elimination phase can sometimes take less than 3 weeks if you have undergone a hydrogen breath testing which aims to identify which particular FODMAPs are the main culprits.

Otherwise, it is likely that you will need to be in this phase for at least 3 weeks to allow your body enough time to adjust.

Phase 2: Reintroduction/Rechallenge the next phase is the reintroduction plan, also called the rechallenge phase. This involves reintroducing the FODMAPs to your diet, one at a time, to see which one triggers your symptoms. For instance, you may reintroduce lactose during the first week. If you show no symptoms and experience no pain, you may then reintroduce fructose as well, and so on. This phase also aims to establish your "threshold level" or the amount of FODMAPs you're able to tolerate.

Once you have identified your triggers, then you'll know which foods you can eat and which ones you should avoid. Remember that you need to remain in a low FODMAP diet throughout this phase. This means, although you tolerate a certain high FODMAP food, you should continue restricting it until the third phase.

Phase 3: Personalization The third phase is also called the "modified low FODMAP diet." In this stage, you still restrict FODMAPs but the type and amount are tailored to your tolerance, as identified during phase 2.

The personalization phase is important because this is where you increase flexibility and variety in your diet. These two qualities are aimed at improving gut health and ensuring long-term compliance.

When your symptoms do not improve...

In the event that you see no improvement in your symptoms during a certain phase or after following all the steps above, here's what you can do:

1. Double check ingredient lists.

Many manufactured foods contain hidden FODMAPs, such as chicken, turkey or beef stock (onions), marinara sauce (garlic and onions), salad dressings (garlic and onions), granola bars (honey, agave syrup, chicory root extract), and gluten-free flour blends (soybean, garbanzo, etc.). Even some supplements contain undeclared FODMAPs such as inulin, mannitol, and sorbitol. These ingredients can prompt symptoms even in low amounts. For this reason, you should always check and recheck labels, and do some research if necessary.

2. Make sure you have correct and accurate FODMAP information.

There are a number of online sources from which you can get a low FODMAP food list. However, most of the lists available on the internet aren't complete. For a validated, more comprehensive list of FODMAP foods and apps, check out the websites of Monash University and King's College London.

3. Consider other life stressors.

Diet isn't the only thing that influences digestive symptoms. Other factors should be taken into consideration as well, most particularly, stress. No matter how strictly you follow your diet, if you're constantly experiencing high levels of stress, then your symptoms will likely persist. If this the case, consider going to therapy as well.

In most cases, following the above process provides significant positive results for people with IBS and IBD. However, according to research, roughly 30% of patients don't respond to a low FODMAP diet. In that event, you may opt for a non-diet-based approach. Discuss alternative options with your doctor.

Low FODMAP Diet Hacks

Adopting a highly restrictive diet can be a challenge, most especially when you're just starting out. So here are a few hacks to help you navigate this complex yet effective diet approach to manage your symptoms and live a happier life.

Choose the low FODMAP cuisines Some cuisines and dietary regimens such as vegetarian, Japanese, Greek, Asian, Ethiopian, and Mediterranean cuisines use low FODMAP products more than others do. You can eat more dishes from these types of cuisines and/or study how to cook them.

Unleash your creative side You have the option to transform your favorite recipes and make them low in FODMAPs. You can substitute high FODMAP ingredients with low FODMAP ones and tweak old-time recipes. And who says you can no longer have flavorful dishes when on a low FODMAP diet? Although you can't use garlic and onion to add flavor to your recipes, you can use many low-FODMAP savory flavorings, herbs and spices as substitute instead. Examples are chives, chili, ginger, fenugreek, mustard seeds, lemongrass, pepper, turmeric, and saffron. Also, while you can't use garlic, you can still get its flavor using garlic-infused oil. And who knows? You may be able to create your very own low FODMAP recipe yourself.

Avoid commercially-prepared sauces Commercially-prepared sauces are usually made using ingredients that have high

FODMAPs. You can still use commercially-made sauces and dips as long as it is indicated in their labels that they are low in FODMAPs. Better yet, you can just make your own sauces so you can be sure that they don't contain any harmful carbohydrates.

When all else fails, opt for the gluten-free option Eating out can be quite difficult when you are in a low FODMAP diet. However, you can make things easier for you by choosing gluten-free products and dishes as these are usually low in FODMAP. Here are other appropriate food choices when dining out:

Cereals and breads made from oats

Tea or coffee with lactose-free milk

Low FODMAP salads, with nuts, seeds, extra-virgin olive oil, and freshly squeezed lemon

Lactose-free yogurt with low-FODMAP fruits on the side

Smoothies and shakes made with low FODMAP fruits and veggies and lactose-free milk

Grilled, roasted, or steamed low FODMAP vegetables

Plain egg, fish, and meat dishes (separate gravies or sauces)

Beef with mustard or chicken/turkey with egg mayonnaise

Popcorn when at the cinema is okay

Sashimi and sushi with wasabi and soy sauce

When travelling, bring a thermos filled with almond milk or lactose-free milk to add to your oatmeal

Knowledge is power The low FODMAP diet can be quite confusing especially if you are just a beginner. Thus, you should not hesitate to whip out your phone and check for answers online if you are unsure whether a food product is low in FODMAPs or not.

Some food products like chickpeas, feta cheese, and bananas contain high amounts of FODMAP in huge servings, but that does not mean that you would have to avoid them altogether. You can still consume products such as these as long as you follow the recommended servings.

Being in a low FODMAP diet doesn't have to be a torture. You can still enjoy scrumptious meals even though you are avoiding some food products. Just be creative in cooking your meals and your low FODMAP journey will surely be a delicious and satisfying one.

How to Practice the Low FODMAP Diet

The low-FODMAP diet aims to remove or reduce foods that are high in FODMAPs from our diet, but it can be a little tricky because there isn't any sure way of measuring the amount of FODMAPs found in foods. Although, it's not impossible. A group of researchers at Monash University in Melbourne, Australia, were the first to conduct a research to observe if a low-FODMAP diet would help relieve the symptoms of IBS and even went further to measure the FODMAP content of a lot of foods through food analysis. Since it's being recommended as a way to manage IBS, I would say that research was a success.

A lot of people would assume that the low-FODMAP diet is like every other diet out there, aim at helping people manage and lose weight, it isn't. It's sole aim is to help people eliminate foods that are high in short-chain carbs from their diet, as a way to reduce recurrent symptoms of IBS. But before jumping head first into the diet as it may seem like a heaven-sent solution to your problem, I would advise you to have a chat with your doctor or dietician about it first because the diet is very restrictive.

Recommended Foods for The Low FODMAP Diet

The biggest dilemma people with IBS face is what to eat. Think about it. When you have a nightmare where you found yourself in a really dark place, for a couple of days, even months, you'll find that you get uncomfortable in dark environments. But what do you do? Will always walk around with a torch? Or do you face your fears? It's the same in this case, we all need food to survive, so you can't totally avoid food for fear of triggering your symptoms. But there's a solution, and I am sure you will be glad to hear it. Along with the elimination and reintroduction phase, it is also very helpful to know the foods recommended for the low-FODMAP diet, because it is sometimes hard to gain relief from IBS symptoms but very easy to trigger them. So, what are they? What are these heaven-sent foods that can give you relief at last?

Low-FODMAP Fruits

I know what you are thinking, how in the clouds do you tell a low-FODMAP fruit from a high-FODMAP fruit? Well, you don't have to go to the lab to get it tested, that's for sure. All you need to know is that low-FODMAP fruits are low in fructans and fructose. With this little information and some research, I am sure you'll learn thats fruits like; oranges, honeydew melons, kiwis, bananas, cantaloupe, lemons, blueberries, pineapples, grapes, strawberries and raspberries are all low-FODMAP and completely acceptable on a low-FODMAP diet.

Most Seeds and Nuts

We all know the nutritional values of nuts and seeds and thankfully, most of them are low-FODMAP. a few of which are; Pecans, chia seeds, macadamia nuts, brazil nuts, pumpkin seeds, pine nuts, sunflower seeds, walnuts, sesame seeds, and peanuts. \

Low-FODMAP Veggies

It may seem a bit overwhelming with the wide variety of vegetables we have, but examples of a few very common low-FODMAP vegetables are; carrots, cabbage, broccoli, eggplant, kale, ginger, okra, radish, seaweed, yam, tomatoes, english and baby spinach, potatoes, cucumbers and fennels.

Most Non-Dairy Milk

Since most dairy milk are notorious for triggering IBS symptoms, here are a few alternatives; coconut milk (in very small amounts, hemp milk, almond milk, and rice milk.

Low-FODMAP Grains

While there are a couple grains that are not accepted on a low-FODMAP diet, others like; quinoa, amaranth, bulgur (in small amounts), oats, brown rice, and spelt are safe because most of them are gluten free.

Some Sweeteners

A lot of sweeteners these days are either high in fructose or fructans or both, and as you know, those are enemies to the low-FODMAP diet. So, what do my fellow compadres with sweet teeth do? Live a life with no sweetness? Waste away and sink deeper into bitter misery? No! We want low-FODMAP sweeteners! We have our pitchforks and torches at the ready, we will do what we must! Fortunately, we won't have to resort to violence, low-FODMAP sweeteners like white sugar, powdered sugar, maple syrup, brown sugar and a couple of artificial sweeteners have jumped in and saved the day.

Tofu and Tempeh

These can serve as great sources of protein for people on the low-FODMAP diet. Vegans can also use them as an alternative for high-FODMAP legumes to make up for their protein requirements.

Fish, Meat And Eggs

Good news! O ye meat and fish lovers! All other non-dairy animal products are acceptable on a low-FODMAP diet. So, you can join in and devour that roasted turkey during Thanksgiving, some chicken wings with friends, barbecued beef with the besties, pork rind on a nice weekend and eggs for breakfast! Hurray! Although, you are advised to avoid processed meats like corned beef and sausages. I am sure you can live with that.

Lactose-Free Dairy Products

The main reason why dairy products are considered high-FODMAP is because they contain lactose. So, if you are in the mood for some yoghurt or ice cream , or you have a bowl of cereal heaped with milk in front of you, you might want to think again.

You don't necessarily have to do without, you can opt for lactose-free options. You can also have some cheeses like parmesan and mozzarella on the diet.

How to Make Life Easier on The Diet?

No diet is easy because you are being drawn out of your comfort zone. Although, it is for the greater good. Even though the low-FODMAP diet can be a bit challenging, here are a few tips to make the diet easy peasy;

Variety is the spice of life; explore new types of food in this diet. Do not just stick to those that you are familiar with. If you eat the same thing over and over again, it will soon get boring and thereby making the diet more difficult to stick to. Challenge yourself to eat a little of everything so that you can make up your daily nutritional needs.

Do not eat too many fruits at a go; I am sure you need no explanation on this one, because too many fruits are high in fructose or fructans or both, so? In this case, less is more.

Do not drink too much alcohol; While it might be fun to club and party to your heart's content, the aftermath is not always pleasant for your bowels. So, have some pity, if not for yourself, but for your poor, abused bowels.

Stay hydrated; Make water your best friend. It helps move stool easier in your bowels. So, drop that soda and take a sip of water. Who knows? You might just be one sip away from sweet relief

Try to space out your meals; A couple of hours between meals is sure to ease your abdominal pain , so wait at least 3-4 hours after each meal or if you can wait, you can make it longer.

Buy seasonal produce; it is highly recommended that you consume only fresh fruits and vegetables, but they tend to be very expensive. So, to minimize cost, you could try buying those that are in season, they are usually cheaper.

Buy only Low-FODMAP certified foods; sometimes you crave the things you used to have, don't worry, it's perfectly normal. When you need pasta, cereals, grains and breads, opt for those that have been certified by the Monash University.

Dietary Modifications

A lot of people with IBD or IBS have one allergy or the other or food intolerance. Some of the most allergens are; shellfish, gluten, dairy, nuts and soy. So, below are a few tips on how to modify the low-FODMAP diet to suit your allergy.

Gluten-free; Although the low-FODMAP diet may contain gluten, you can totally omit those foods from your diet without any harm. So, instead of rye or barley, you can use quinoa or brown rice instead.

Vegan; Vegans normally rely on foods like split peas, beans and lentils as a source of protein, but these foods are high-FODMAP, which makes it very difficult for vegans to get enough protein on a low-FODMAP diet. To make up for that, foods like quinoa, tempeh, tofu, seeds and nuts are recommended.

Children; Children have a lot of nutritional needs, that is why many diets aren't recommended for children, and the low-FODMAP diet isn't an exception. Research hasn't yet been made in regards to the safety of a low-FODMAP diet for children, so if your child has IBS related symptoms, you might want to talk to a pediatrician. If a supervised Low-FODMAP diet is suggested, then you might want to try it, only until your child feels better.

Soy-free; foods containing soy are not allowed on a low-FODMAP diet, so if you use soy as a source of protein, you might want to try something else. Animal products or nuts are also good options.

Pregnancy; No research has been done as of yet as regards to a low-FODMAP diet in pregnancy, so it is not recommended. Although if you have any IBS related symptoms in pregnancy, you might want to avoid or reduce your intake of the foods that you are sensitive to.

Dairy-free; The low-FODMAP diet is mostly dairy free, but to make it completely so, you should skip the lactose-free products and soft-cheeses and opt for Low-FODMAP non-dairy milk instead.

Vegetarians; Vegetarians can consume foods containing dairy products, unlike their vegan counterparts, but since there are restrictions on dairy products for the low-FODMAP diet, vegetarians are advised to go for lactose-free dairy or non-dairy products and also consume enough low-FODMAP proteins.

Allergen-Friendly; Adopting an allergen-friendly low-FODMAP diet can be really challenging, but not impossible. If you are allergic to some foods such as shellfish or tree nuts, just avoid them, they won't affect how you react to other foods.

Is the Low-FODMAP Diet Plan Right for You?

If you suffer from IBS and symptoms of chronic digestive distress, then you are likely all too aware that your food choices significantly impact the presence and severity of your symptoms. Before the FODMAP diet was discovered, narrowing down the foods that caused the worst symptoms was a complicated guessing game at best. Even today, many people still suffer unnecessarily from painful symptoms that can be eased with the correct knowledge. In fact, it is estimated that only ten percent of the people who suffer from symptoms of IBS actually seek medical help. This means that there is an incredible number of people out there, suffering quietly with painful digestive issues.

Even those of us who do seek help for our symptoms are often led down a path of nutritional advice that can be more harmful than healing. To be fair, the varied symptoms and severity of IBS can make it difficult to easily recognize and treat. For example, many people with IBS deal with chronic diarrhea or constipation. If you were to go to a doctor and describe just these symptoms, you might be told to add more soluble fiber to your diet. Soluble fiber is great, and beneficial to your health, unless you have IBS where certain forms of it can make your symptoms worse. Foods like apples and fiber fortified wheat breads are excellent sources of soluble fiber. They are also on the high-FODMAP food list. Essentially, the very foods that you are eating to ease your symptoms are only making them worse.

This is in part because as part of their education, doctors are taught to look for the simplest explanation first, because often, it is the correct diagnosis. In many cases, this is beneficial for both the doctor and the patient. Is it necessary to go through the process of and costs of sophisticated diagnostic tests if your issue can be easily addressed without going through all of that? This philosophy saves doctors and patients time and allows physicians to begin treatment faster. The problem is when the treatment doesn't work, and you go back looking for more answers.

Chapter 2: Overview of Fodmaps: what is IBS, SIBO, and IBD.

IBS and IBD are often confused with each other because they sound almost alike. While they share the same name and a few similar symptoms, these two disorders have distinct differences and require different treatments.

IBS, or Irritable Bowel Syndrome, isn't classified as a real disease, rather, it is a functional disorder primarily characterized by abdominal pain and altered bowel movements. Other symptoms include gas, bloating, cramps, constipation, and diarrhea. With this condition, the digestive tract appears to be physically normal but its proper functioning is in some ways disrupted. IBS affects up to 15% of the world population and is more common in women than in men.

On the other hand, IBD, or Inflammatory Bowel Disease, is an autoimmune condition marked by chronic intestinal swelling or inflammation. It is a structural disease caused by an underlying physical damage in the gut. Unlike IBS, IBD manifests physical changes in the digestive tract as a result of the recurrent inflammation. It causes the same symptoms as IBS, with the addition of:

extreme fatigue

eye inflammation

joint pain

intestinal scarring

rectal bleeding

This condition may also cause long-term health concerns such as micronutrient deficiencies, malnutrition, and weight loss. The most common types of IBD include ulcerative colitis, indeterminate colitis, and Chron's disease.

Both IBS and IBD can trigger urgent bowel movements. Also, both conditions can negatively impact a person's life as they can lead to high healthcare costs, frequent absenteeism from school or work, and poor quality of life in general.

Causes of IBS and IBD

People with IBS don't show any clinical signs of a digestive disease and they often have normal clinical test results. For this reason, the exact cause of IBS remains unclear. However, it has been linked to the immune system and the way by which the muscles move the food through the stomach. There are certain triggers that can aggravate the symptoms, such as infections, hormonal changes, stress, and certain foods.

For IBD patients, the ongoing inflammation in their gut (which results from the autoimmune response of the cells) can cause ulcers (sores) and bleeding. In turn, this causes severe digestive stress and pain. It can also lead to symptoms like fatigue and fever by exacerbating the immune system.

Role of Stress Contrary to common belief, IBS is not a psychological condition. However, it appears to aggravate with stress. Hence, stress reduction techniques such as meditation, yoga, regular exercise, and talk therapy may help manage its symptoms. This is supported by a study published in The American Journal of Gastroenterology which showed reduced severity of IBS symptoms after 8 weeks of mindfulness meditation.

IBD was once believed to be triggered by stress. However, there is no evidence to support this claim. In any case, IBD patients shouldn't feel like or think that they brought the illness upon themselves, which seems to be the case sometimes due to the social stigmas associated with the said condition.

Diagnosing IBS

IBS can be quite difficult to diagnose and often requires multiple diagnostic tests. But first, doctors must rule out any serious conditions like celiac disease, small intestinal bacterial growth, or IBD. Once that's done, the diagnosis is done based on stool patterns and symptoms.

Doctors may also use the "Rome criteria" to determine whether or not you have IBS. According to said criteria, you may have IBS if you've been experiencing stomach pains for at least once a day per week for the past 3 months, and the pain meets at least 2 of the following:

it is coupled with a bowel movement;

your bowel movements occur less or more often when the pain starts; and

your stool looks different when the pain begins to occur.

As the doctor deems necessary, other clinical tests may be conducted after using the above standards for a more accurate diagnosis of IBS.

Treatment Presently, there is no known cure for IBS and IBD, but there are various ways to control the symptoms and manage the conditions. These include special diets, medications, and supplements.

Diet: Following a low FODMAP diet is one of the easiest, most promising ways of controlling the symptoms of IBS and IBD. 3 out of 4 people who stick to this diet report that their symptoms and the quality of their life have improved since making the switch. Although it isn't an actual cure, low FODMAP diet, along with some lifestyle changes, greatly helps with the overall management of the disorders.

Medications: IBD is typically treated with certain medications that target inflammation in the gut, and these may vary depending on the diagnosis. The doctor may also prescribe medicines for constipation or diarrhea if the patient needs more relief. However, to treat and prevent inflammation remains the primary goal.

IBS can be controlled by taking intestinal antispasmodics like dicyclomine (Bentyl) and hyoscyamine (Levsin). Powerful medications for IBD often don't work for IBS, so it's important to be certain of your condition.

Supplements: Experts are also studying the potential of probiotics as treatment for the disorders. However, this area of research is still evolving. Hopefully, probiotic supplements that specifically target IBS and IBD will one day be developed.

Other methods that can be helpful include acupuncture, relaxation training, hypnotherapy, and stress management. If your condition is causing you too much stress and is already affecting your social life, you may also consider counseling and joining support groups.

Many people suffering from irritation bowel disease, and every other form of digestive disorders are usually susceptible to the negative impacts of foods that are high in FODMAPs. The result of eating such foods often makes a person feel a high level of discomfort that doctors and dietitians had to make studies into any possible means of treating the result. Aside from the foods arousing your IBS symptoms, it makes the gut uncomfortable. This shows that regardless of how tasty the food might be; it will be useless to the gut. You can live a healthy life. The studies done on the effects of foods that are high in FODMAPs on the gut has led to a new diet that helps to fight off the triggers to the IBS symptoms and give a person a better dietary lifestyle that is not detrimental to his or her health. The new diet is a low-FODMAP diet that helps to deal with the symptoms that are made to come out whenever foods that are high FODMAPs are eaten.

Chapter 3: Everything You need to know about how digestion works.

We are all different from each other, and as such, our digestive systems are highly different. Over time, our reactions to some foods will change, it could be due to age, the overall health of one's digestive system, environment or lifestyle. You might notice that you have no problem with certain foods in your youth, but as you age, you will notice that you become more intolerant. Sometimes, you might not even have a problem with a certain food today, but it may cause you extreme discomfort the next day. None till date knows why these dramatic changes occur because the human digestive system is very complex. Amazing right? If you ask me, I'd say we've barely scratched the surface where the digestive system is concerned. I mean, how can we claim to fully understand something so amazingly complex?

It might sound a little bit gross but I am sure you didn't know that your lower digestive tract is home to many bacteria, both good and bad, and there is a definite cycle in motion on the microbial level. When you are stressed or Ill, the medicines you take all affect your gut bacteria, because they feed off of what you eat.

But if you find yourself frequently dealing with digestive problems, maybe chronic gas, constipation, diarrhea, bloating and abdominal (which are all symptoms of IBS), then you are probably sensitive to high-FODMAP foods.

How FODMAPs Affect the Gut

When FODMAPs are introduced into the digestive system, they increase the production of intestinal gas and cause fluid changes. Small FODMAP molecules, exert an osmotic effect in the intestines which is the reason why fluids are drawn into the bowels, and gut bacteria waste no time working on FODMAPs which causes them to ferment and produce gas and as a result, the bowels get distended, which is why you tend to get bloated or have abdominal pain. It also alters the way the muscles of the bowels contract. When peristalsis (forward movement) is increased, it can cause diarrhea for some and constipation in others. For example, fructose can draw twice as much fluids into your bowels than glucose(which is not a FODMAP) because it is "osmotically active" .

A lot of people are of the misconception that the inability to break down FODMAPS happens in only people with IBS, which is a very wrong assumption because even perfectly healthy people find it difficult to breakdown FODMAPs, which is perfectly normal. Although, it is only in people with IBS that symptoms are easily triggered, which may be as a result of;

The type of bacteria in the bowels; when there is an overgrowth of bacteria in the small intestine, it results in a condition called "SIBO" or "small intestine bacterial overgrowth" which leads to excessive gas production in the bowels, which as you know, results in bloating, abdominal pain, distension etc.

The manner in which the muscles of the bowels respond to distension; this may result in fast or slow passage of stool in the bowels. The gut is really sensitive, so it easily picks up on changes or any alterations in the gut environment and interacts with the immune system and nervous system in response to these changes. Which means people with IBS have lower pain tolerance when their bowels are distended than healthy adults.

These two factors are what determine a person's reaction to FODMAPs, but there are those who aren't sensitive to FODMAPs, so they won't react the same way a person with IBS will, even with the factors listed above. This is thought to be as a result of a condition called colonic hypersensitivity, which is pretty common in people with IBS. So, it's not like there is anything special about those who do not have colonic hypersensitivity, they are just lucky! Because these we are all unable to breakdown these short-chain carbs, they just bother the unlucky ones. But the question is why? Like I said before, it's mostly due to a person's hypersensitivity to certain changes to the gut environment, certain illnesses or stress.

Chapter 4: The importance of fodmap with the intestine

Effects of FODMAPs on our Gut – Fluid Changes & Production of Intestinal Gas

In our small and large intestines, the small FODMAP molecules use an osmotic effect, which means that more fluid is strained into our bowel. FODMAPs are likewise quickly inflamed by colonic microflora-producing gas. This increase in fluid and gas swells our bowel. It will cause the feeling of swelling and abdominal aching or distress, and disturbs how the muscles in the wall of our bowel contract. This may cause amplified advancing movement (peristalsis) which can lead to diarrhea, but in some people, can cause constipation.

The means by which the muscles of the bowel reply (motility) to the swelling: They can result in faster or slower passageway through the gut.

The gut is "oversensitive" to variations in the gut setting and to relations with the nervous system & immune system in the digestive tract: This means that IBS people are more likely to distinguish pain at a lesser threshold when swelling of the bowel is present, likened to healthy adults.

The kind of bacteria in our bowel: The bowel bacteria could yield greater amounts of gas, or there could be amplified bacterial numbers in the small intestines (called small intestinal bacterial overgrowth - or SIBO) so that now more gas is formed in the small bowel. Swelling of the small bowel will cause amplified abdominal uneasiness, distension, & bloating.

This is especially true for people who suffer from IBS, FGID, SIBO and IBDs. Not only are there specific nutritional concerns that might need to be addressed, a qualified professional can also help you identify other factors that should be considered before embarking on a low-FODMAP plan. People who have very inflexible preferences regarding food choices, those who have suffered from or are at risk of eating disorders, those who have dietary restrictions due to other medical conditions and those who already eat a generally low-FODMAP diet should seek additional medical advice to discuss starting, and possibly modifying, this plan to meet your health and nutritional needs.

Recognize that eliminating all potential triggers at once means that you will be temporarily changing not only your dietary habits, but quite possibly your lifestyle as well. One of the downfalls of any diet is the period of adjustment where your body is adjusting to the changes while your mind is still stuck in old patterns of thinking and behavior. Add to it that sometimes there is a period of detoxification where you might notice some new uncomfortable symptoms for a few days. This is especially true if following a low-FODMAP plan drastically changes the types of foods that you typically consume daily.

Starting out on the low-FODMAP plan should not be combined with a change of medications, vitamins or supplements. The reason for this is quite simple. If you are changing or adding a medication, how do you know if the effects on your digestive health are really from the elimination of FODMAPs or from another source? It is best to start the low-FODMAP plan when everything else in your daily routine is stable.

When you decide to commit to a low-FODMAP plan, you really need to go all in, and give 100% of your effort. Since the low-FODMAP plan is an elimination diet, if you introduce just one of the eliminated foods, even just a bite, you need to start over from scratch to achieve the most accurate results.

Think about it for a minute. You have diligently committed to eating only low-FODMAP foods for the past two weeks, and you are starting to notice some changes in how you feel. Then let's say you go out to dinner and in front of you is a basket of fresh from the oven rolls, served with an irresistible honey butter. The smell is intoxicating and your dinner companions are enjoying the treat with abandon. You think to yourself, could one or two bites really hurt? For the sake of the elimination diet, the answer is yes. With just that one bite, you are ingesting multiple FODMAPs. You may or may not have an increase in symptoms from that roll, but if you do, how will you know which of the FODMAPs are to blame. The only solution at this point is to start over by clearing your system of all FODMAPs.

Now that you are mentally prepared to start the low-FODMAP plan, let's get down to the more practical aspects and tips for success.

Chapter 5: 7-Day Diet Plans

DAY	BREAKFAST	LUNCH	DINNER	DESSERT
1.	Salmon Omelet with Spinach	Creamy Stuffed Potatoes	Low FODMAP Potato Salad	No-Bake Energy Bars
2.	Chocolate Chia Breakfast Bowl	Asian Chicken and Rice Bowl	Lemon Ginger Chicken and Rice Soup	Frozen Yogurt Bark with Berries
3.	Blueberry French Toast Bake	Brie Caprese Style Polenta	Gluten-free Chicken & Vegetable Pie	Peanut Butter Oatmeal Chocolate Chip Cookies
4.	Velvety Scrambled Eggs	Salmon and Spinach	Pad Thai With Shrimps	Blueberry Crumble

5.	Potato Salad with Quail's Eggs	Spaghetti Bolognese	Coconut Chicken Rice Noodle	Instant Banana Pudding
6.	Pumpkin Pancakes	Tuna Fried Rice	Beef and Vegetable Stir Fry with Oyster Sauce	Chocolate-Orange-Raspberry Cupcakes
7.	Delicious Paprika Potatoes	Tuna Noodle Casserole	Chicken and Rice	Baked Brie with Cranberry Chutney and Caramelized Pecans

Chapter 6: Breakfast

Salmon Omelet with Spinach

Cooking Time: 15 minutes

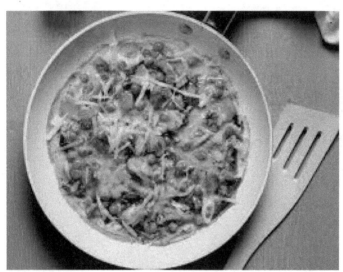

Servings: 2

Ingredients:

6 large eggs

8 pieces cherry tomato

1 ½ tablespoons almond milk

3 tablespoons fresh parsley, chopped

1/8 teaspoon paprika

60 g spinach, shredded

3 teaspoons canola oil

3 teaspoons sesame oil

210 g canned plain pink salmon, drained

Salt and pepper to taste

Direction:

Whisk the eggs together with milk. Sprinkle with salt and pepper to taste.

Place a frying pan with canola oil over medium-low heat.

Pour the egg mixture into the pan and season with paprika. Cook for about 8 minutes.

Flip the omelet and cook until firm.

Put salmon, sesame oil and parsley in a small bowl. Mix well.

Transfer the salmon mixture into a frying pan and heat it over medium flame.

Add spinach into the salmon mixture and cook until wilted.

Put the omelet on a plate with the salmon mixture and cherry tomatoes on top. Sprinkle with black pepper, if desired.

Nutrition: 534 calories, 5.9 g sugars, 460.5 mg calcium, 9.5 g saturates, 5.3 mg iron, 49.3 g protein, 0.8 g salt, 8.3 g carbohydrates and 1.9 g fiber.

Chocolate Chia Breakfast Bowl

Cooking Time: 3 minutes

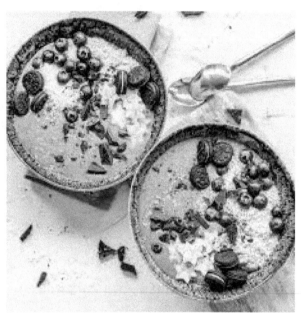

Servings: 1

Ingredients:

125 milliliters almond milk

3 tablespoons chia seeds

1 ½ teaspoon pure maple syrup

¾ tablespoon cocoa powder, unsweetened

½ teaspoon vanilla extract

Direction:

Put milk, vanilla extract, maple syrup and cocoa powder in a small bowl. Using a fork, stir the ingredients together until there are no more lumps.

Add chia seeds and mix well.

Cover the bowl and place it in the refrigerator. Let it cool for about 6 hours or overnight.

Break up any lumps that formed in the mixture. Serve with fruit of your choice.

Nutrition: 315 calories, 347.6 mg calcium, 10.9 g fat, 3.5 mg iron, 1.5 g saturates, 23.1 g sugars, 0.1-gram salt, 7 g protein, 14.3 g fiber and 52.4 g carbohydrates.

Blueberry French Toast Bake

Cooking Time: 45 minutes

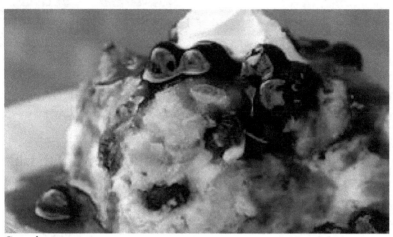

Servings: 12

Ingredients:

500 g spelt sourdough or wheat bread, cubed

167 g brown sugar

150 g fresh blueberries

3 teaspoons vanilla extract

8 pieces large eggs

½ teaspoon nutmeg, ground

1 teaspoon cinnamon, ground

563 milliliters almond milk

70 g plain flour, gluten-free

70 g cold butter, cubed

Direction:

Use butter to grease an oven-proof dish.

Spread blueberries and bread cubes evenly in the oven-proof dish. Set aside.

Put eggs, ½ teaspoon cinnamon, 100 g brown sugar, milk, nutmeg and vanilla extract in a large bowl. Stir the mixture until no lumps remains.

Pour the mixture evenly over the blueberries and bread cubes. Cover the dish with a plastic wrap and leave it in the refrigerator for 3 hours or overnight.

Set the oven to 180 degrees Celsius. In the meantime, take out the oven dish from the refrigerator and set aside.

Combine the flour with the remaining amounts of sugar and cinnamon in a medium bowl. Mix well.

Add about three-fourths of the butter into the mixture and stir until it becomes quite lumpy. Crumble the remaining amount of butter.

Distribute the flour mixture and crumbled butter evenly on top of the bread mixture in the oven dish.

Bake the bread mixture in the oven until the top becomes golden brown in color. This should take about 40 to 50 minutes.

Serve with pure maple syrup or fruit of your choice.

Nutrition: 323 calories, 121.8 mg calcium, 10.2 g fat, 2.7 mg iron, 2.2 g saturates, 19.6 g sugars, 0.4 g salt, 10.4 g protein, 1.5 g fiber and 46.8 g carbohydrates.

Velvety Scrambled Eggs

Cooking Time: 20 minutes

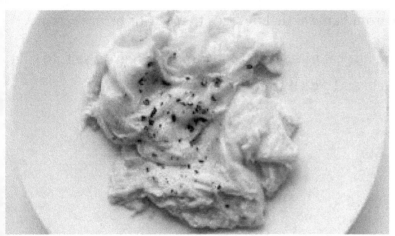

Servings: 1

Ingredients:

2 large eggs

Butter

6 tablespoons single cream

Direction:

Lightly beat eggs together with cream. Season with salt.

Melt butter in a pan for a minute. Add egg mixture and let it cook slightly for 20 seconds without stirring.

Stir egg mixture using a wooden spoon and allow to cook for another 10 minutes. Repeat Direction until eggs are set but still soft.

Remove from flame and allow eggs to rest. Stir before serving.

Nutrition: 254 calories, 4 g carbohydrates, 0.6-gram salt, 19 g fat, 18 g protein and 7 g saturates.

Potato Salad with Quail's Eggs

Cooking Time: 30 minutes

Servings: 1

Ingredients:

4 quail's eggs

1 anchovy, chopped

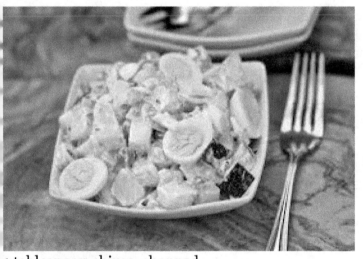

1 tablespoon chives, chopped

100 g green beans

1 tablespoon parsley, chopped

100 g potatoes, quartered

Juice of ½ lemon

Direction:

Allow water in a medium pan to a simmer. Cook quail's eggs for 2 minutes. Once done, place eggs in a bowl of cold water.

Place green beans in the hot water. Simmer for 4 minutes. Transfer to a bowl of cold water. After cooling, peel eggs and slice in half.

Put potatoes in the hot water. Cook for 15 minutes then drain excess water once potatoes are tender. Set aside to cool.

Add the green beans, chives, anchovy, parsley and lemon juice. Toss to mix.

Serve with eggs on top.

Nutrition: 174 calories, 4 g sugars, 0.5-gram salt, 5 g fat, 9 g protein, 2 g saturates, 5 g fiber and 20 g carbohydrates.

Pumpkin Pancakes

Cooking Time: 20 minutes:

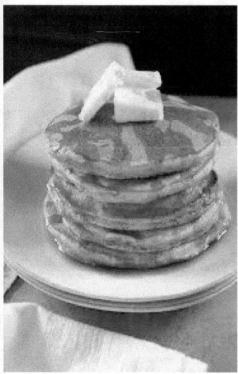

Servings: 1

Ingredients:

½ firm banana, mashed

½ teaspoon pumpkin pie spice

¼ cup pumpkin puree

½ teaspoon vanilla

1 large egg

¼ teaspoon baking powder

2 tablespoons coconut flour

Direction:

Combine pumpkin and banana together in a bowl. Mix well.

Add remaining ingredients. Stir well until smooth.

Pour mixture in a pan. Cook over medium heat in oil for 5 minutes on each side. Repeat Direction for the remaining mixture.

Nutrition: 231 calories, 9 g protein, 7 g fat, 8 g fiber and 35 g carbohydrates.

Quinoa Breakfast Bowl

Cooking Time: 25 minutes

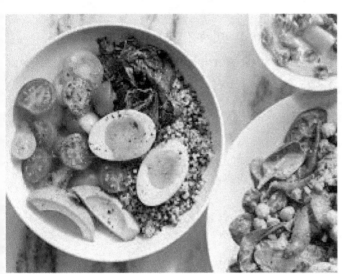

Servings: 4

Ingredients:

1 cup quinoa

1 cup coconut, toasted

2 cups water

Juice of 1/4 lime

Direction:

Place quinoa in a pan with water.

Bring the water to a boil. Reduce heat to medium-low.

Simmer for 20 minutes. Add coconut and drizzle with lime juice. Mix well.

Serve with fruits and nuts of choice.

Nutrition: 228 calories, 5 mg iron, 9.3 g fat, 24 mg calcium, 6.2 g saturates, 4.8 g fiber, 6.7 g protein, 0.01-gram salt, 1.3 g sugars and 30.5 g carbohydrates

Delicious Paprika Potatoes

Servings: 4

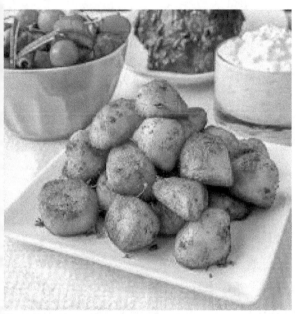

Preparation time: 5 minutes

Cooking time: 30 minutes

1 lb baby potatoes, quartered

2 tbsp coconut oil, melted

1 tbsp olive oil

¼ tsp rosemary, crushed

½ tsp thyme

2 tbsp paprika

Pepper

Salt

Direction:

Preheat the oven to 425 F/ 218 C.

Place potatoes on a baking tray and sprinkle with paprika, rosemary, thyme, pepper, and salt.

Drizzle with oil and melted coconut oil.

Bake in preheated oven for 30 minutes. Shake after every 10 minutes.

Serve and enjoy.

Nutrition: Calories: 138; Total Fat: 7.4g; Saturated Fat: 6g; Protein: 3.6g; Carbs: 16.9g; Fiber: 4.3g; Sugar: 0.4g

Raspberry Scones

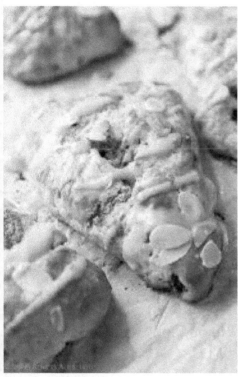

Servings: 8

Preparation time: 15 minutes

Cooking time: 13 minutes

¼ cup raspberries, diced

1 tbsp lemon juice

1 tsp lemon zest

2 tbsp coconut oil, melted

6 tbsp almond milk

2 tsp baking powder

3 tbsp brown sugar

2 tbsp cornstarch

¼ cup brown rice flour

½ cup almond flour

¾ cup oat flour

½ tsp salt

Direction:

In a mixing bowl, mix together almond flour, oat flour, baking powder, brown sugar, and salt.

In another bowl, stir together almond milk, lemon juice, lemon zest, and oil.

Add wet mixture to the dry mixture and stir until well combined.

Add raspberries and fold well and place dough in the fridge for 1 hour.

Preheat the oven to 350 F/ 180 C.

Spray a baking tray with cooking spray and set aside.

Remove dough from fridge and roll dough into a ½-inch thick circle.

Slice dough into eight triangles and place onto a prepared baking tray.

Bake in preheated oven for 13 minutes.

Serve and enjoy.

Nutrition: Calories: 171; Total Fat: 10.3g; Saturated Fat: 5.8g; Protein: 3.3g; Carbs: 18g; Fiber: 2.4g; Sugar: 4.2g

Healthy Oat Cookies

Servings: 3

Preparation time: 10 minutes

Cooking time: 12 minutes

½ cup oats

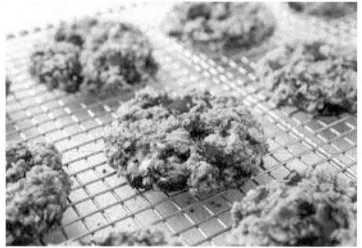

1 tsp walnuts, chopped

1 tsp dried cranberries

1 tsp almonds, sliced

1 tsp chocolate chips

1 banana

Direction:

Preheat the oven to 350 F/ 180 C.

Spray a baking tray with cooking spray and set aside.

Add banana in a bowl and mash using a fork.

Add remaining ingredients to the bowl and mix well.

Make cookies from mixture and place on a prepared baking tray and bake for 12 minutes.

Serve and enjoy.

Nutrition: Calories: 103; Total Fat: 2.2g; Saturated Fat: 0.5g; Protein: 2.7g; Carbs: 19.2g; Fiber: 2.6g; Sugar: 5.6g

Blueberry Bars

Servings: 9

Preparation time: 10 minutes

Cooking time: 25 minutes

Top layer:

¼ cup almond milk

½ tsp cinnamon

1 ½ tbsp chia seeds

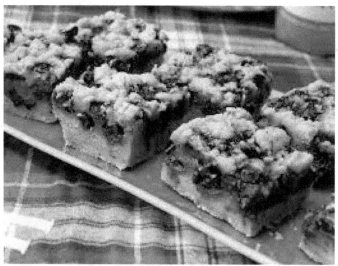

3 tbsp walnuts, chopped

¼ cup pumpkin seeds

½ cup oats

1 cup blueberries

Bottom layer:

2 tsp coconut oil

½ tsp cinnamon

1 scoop vanilla protein powder

2 bananas

4 tbsp maple syrup

2 cups oats

¼ tsp salt

Direction:

Preheat the oven to 350 F/ 180 C.

Spray a 9*9-inch baking dish with cooking spray and set aside.

Add all ingredients of the bottom layer into the food processor and process for 1 minute and transfer into the prepared dish. Spread mixture evenly and bake in preheated oven for 10 minutes.

Add all top layer ingredients into the mixing bowl and mix well.

Remove baking dish from oven and top with bowl mixture. Spread mixture evenly and bake for 15 minutes more.

Remove from oven and let it cool completely.

Cut into squares and serve.

Nutrition: Calories: 221; Total Fat: 7.9g; Saturated Fat: 3g; Protein: 8.4g; Carbs: 31.5g; Fiber: 4.1g; Sugar: 10.7g

Tofu Scramble

Servings: 2

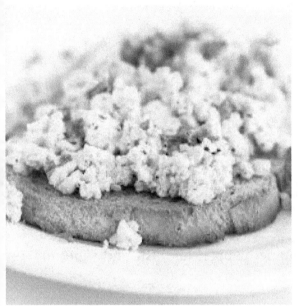

Preparation time: 10 minutes

Cooking time: 7 minutes

½ block firm tofu, crumbled

¼ cup Alfalfa sprouts

1 tbsp chives, chopped

1 tbsp coriander, chopped

¼ tsp ground cumin

1 tbsp turmeric

1 cup spinach

1 tbsp olive oil

1 medium tomato, chopped

¼ cup zucchini, chopped

Pepper

Salt

Direction:

Heat oil in a pan over medium heat.

Add tomato, zucchini, and spinach to the pan and sauté for 2 minutes.

Add tofu, cumin, turmeric, pepper, and salt and sauté for 4-5 minutes.

Top with Alfalfa sprouts, chives, and coriander.

Serve and enjoy.

Nutrition: Calories: 107; Total Fat: 8.6g; Saturated Fat: 1.4g; Protein: 3.5g; Carbs: 6.4g; Fiber: 2.2g; Sugar: 2.2g

Banana Oat Breakfast Cookies

Servings: 1

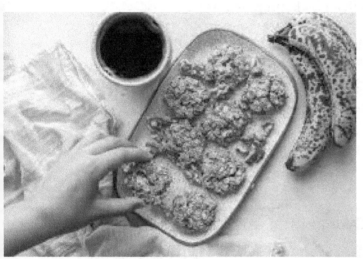

Preparation time: 5 minutes

Cooking time: 12 minutes

½ cup oats

1 tbsp chocolate chips

1 tbsp peanut butter

1 banana

Pinch of salt

Direction:

Preheat the oven to 350 F/ 180 C.

Spray a baking tray with cooking spray. Set aside.

Add banana in a bowl and mash using a fork.

Add remaining ingredients and stir well to combine.

Spoon dollops of batter onto a prepared baking tray and bake for 10-12 minutes.

Serve and enjoy.

Nutrition: Calories: 410; Total Fat: 14g; Saturated Fat: 4.5g; Protein: 11.5g; Carbs: 64g; Fiber: 8.5g; Sugar: 21.8g

Breakfast Smoothie Bowl

Servings: 1

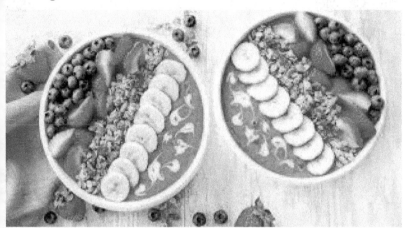

Preparation time: 5 minutes

Cooking time: 5 minutes

1 tbsp maple syrup

½ cup almond milk

1 cup baby spinach

¾ cup pineapple chunks

1/3 banana

Direction:

Add all ingredients into the blender and blend until smooth.

Pour blended mixture into the bowl and top with your favorite toppings and serve.

Nutrition: Calories: 432; Total Fat: 29g; Saturated Fat: 25g; Protein: 4g; Carbs: 46.4g; Fiber: 6.1g; Sugar: 33g

Baked Oatmeal

Servings: 1

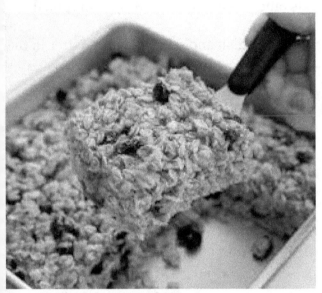

Preparation time: 5 minutes

Cooking time: 15 minutes

½ cup oats

1 tbsp peanut butter

½ banana

¼ cup almond milk

Pinch of salt

Direction:

Preheat the oven to 350 F/ 180 C.

Add banana in a bowl and mash using a fork.

Add almond milk, oats, and salt and mix until well combined.

Pour batter in a small baking dish and spoon peanut butter in the center of mixture.

Place in preheated oven and bake for 15 minutes.

Serve and enjoy.

Nutrition: Calories: 440; Total Fat: 25.2g; Saturated Fat: 14.9g; Protein: 11.4g; Carbs: 47.7g; Fiber: 7.9g; Sugar: 11.1g

Millet Porridge

Servings: 4

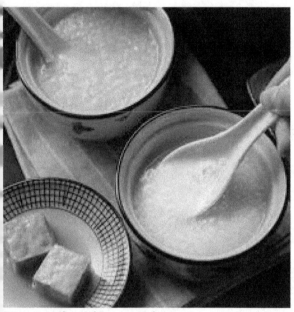

Preparation time: 5 minutes

Cooking time: 25 minutes

2/3 cup hulled millet

1 ½ cups water

2 cups almond milk

Pinch of salt

Direction:

Add millet, water, almond milk, and salt in a saucepan and bring to boil.

Turn heat to low and simmer for 25 minutes.

Serve and enjoy.

Nutrition: Calories: 396; Total Fat: 29.9g; Saturated Fat: 25.4g; Protein: 6.7g; Carbs: 30.6g; Fiber: 8g; Sugar: 4g

Quick Quinoa Porridge

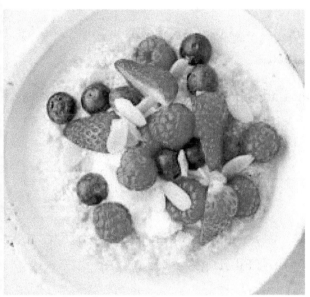

Preparation time: 5 minutes

Cooking time: 2 minutes

2/3 cup quinoa

1 tbsp maple syrup

2 tbsp peanut butter, creamy

½ tsp vanilla

1 cup unsweetened almond milk

1 cup water

Pinch of salt

Direction:

Add milk, vanilla, water, and salt in a saucepan and bring to boil over high heat.

Turn heat to medium and add quinoa. Stir well and cook for 1 minute or until thickened.

Remove from heat and add maple syrup and peanut butter and stir well.

Serve and enjoy.

Nutrition: Calories: 235; Total Fat: 8.8g; Saturated Fat: 1.5g; Protein: 8.3g; Carbs: 31.6g; Fiber: 3.6g; Sugar: 5.1g

Almond Cranberry Oatmeal

Servings: 1

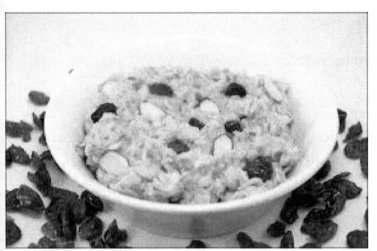

Preparation time: 5 minutes

Cooking time: 10 minutes

½ cup rolled oats

1 ½ tbsp cranberry sauce

½ tsp cinnamon

1 tbsp almond butter

½ cup water

½ cup almond milk

Direction:

Add oats, water, and almond milk in a saucepan and cook over medium-high heat until thickened.

Remove from heat and add cinnamon and almond butter and stir well.

Top with cranberry sauce and serve.

Nutrition: Calories: 538; Total Fat: 40.3g; Saturated Fat: 26.5g; Protein: 11.6g; Carbs: 39.2g; Fiber: 9.4g; Sugar: 5.5g

Chocolate Overnight Oats

Servings: 2

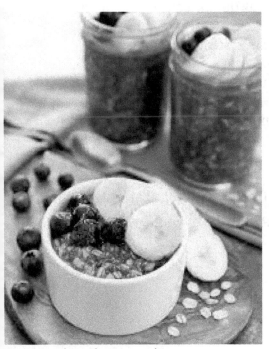

Preparation time: 5 minutes

Cooking time: 5 minutes

1 cup almond milk

1 cup rolled oats

¼ tsp cinnamon

1 tbsp cocoa powder

2/3 banana

2 tbsp walnuts, chopped

Direction:

Add banana in a mixing bowl and mash using a fork.

Add cinnamon and cocoa powder and stir until smooth.

Add almond milk and oats and stir to combine.

Cover bowl and place in the refrigerator for overnight.

Stir well and top with walnuts and serve.

Nutrition: Calories: 521; Total Fat: 36.4g; Saturated Fat: 26.3g; Protein: 10.9g; Carbs: 45.8g; Fiber: 9.3g; Sugar: 9.4g

Cookie Dough Oatmeal

Servings: 2

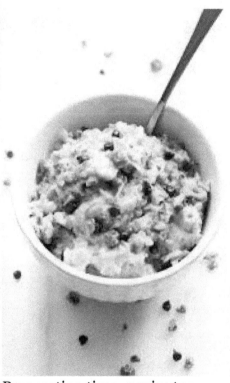

Preparation time: 5 minutes

Cooking time: 5 minutes

1 tbsp chocolate chips

4 tbsp walnuts, chopped

1 tbsp maple syrup

½ tsp vanilla

1 ¼ cup almond milk

1/8 tsp nutmeg

½ tsp cinnamon

2 tbsp chia seeds

1 cup rolled oats

Pinch of salt

Direction:

Add oats, nutmeg, cinnamon, chia seeds, and salt in a bowl and mix well.

Add almond milk, maple syrup, walnuts, and vanilla and stir well.

Cover and place in the refrigerator for overnight.

Add chocolate chips and stir well.

Serve and enjoy.

Nutrition: Calories: 690; Total Fat: 51.6g; Saturated Fat: 34.1g; Protein: 14.6g; Carbs: 49.6g; Fiber: 9g; Sugar: 14.4g

Turmeric Pineapple Smoothie

Servings: 1

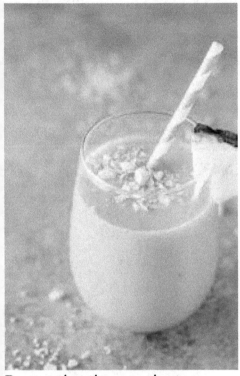

Preparation time: 5 minutes

Cooking time: 5 minutes

½ cup pineapple chunks

¼ tsp ground ginger

¼ tsp turmeric

2 tbsp protein powder

1/3 banana

¾ cup almond milk

Direction:

Add all ingredients into the blender and blend until smooth.

Serve and enjoy.

Nutrition: Calories: 514; Total Fat: 43.2g; Saturated Fat: 38.1g; Protein: 10.1g; Carbs: 30.5g; Fiber: 6.3g; Sugar: 19g

Almond Breakfast Granola

Servings: 12 Preparation time: 10 minutes

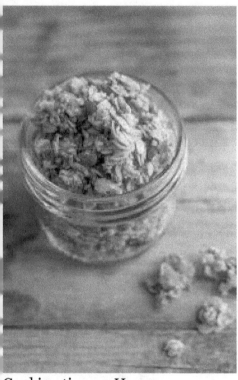

Cooking time: 2 Hours

3 ½ cups rolled oats

½ tbsp vanilla

¼ cup olive oil

½ cup granulated sugar

½ cup water

½ cup almonds, sliced

¼ tsp salt

Direction:

Preheat the oven to 200 F/ 93 C.

Spray a baking tray with cooking spray and line with parchment paper and set aside.

In a mixing bowl, mix together almonds and oats.

Add water, sugar, and salt in a saucepan and cook over medium heat until sugar is dissolved.

Remove from heat and add vanilla and oil and stir well. Pour into the oats mixture and stir to combine.

Spread mixture onto a prepared baking tray and bake for 2 hours or until completely dry.

Allow to cool completely then serve.

Nutrition: Calories: 182; Total Fat: 7.7g; Saturated Fat: 1g; Protein: 4g; Carbs: 25.4g; Fiber: 2.9g; Sugar: 8.8g

Healthy Green Breakfast Smoothie

Servings: 1

Preparation time: 5 minutes

Cooking time: 5 minutes

1 tsp maple syrup

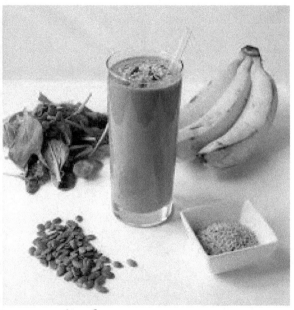

2 cups spinach

¼ cup strawberries

1/3 cup pineapple

½ banana

1 cup almond milk

Direction:

Add all ingredients into the blender and blend until smooth.

Serve and enjoy.

Nutrition: Calories: 675; Total Fat: 57.8g; Saturated Fat: 50.9g; Protein: 8.4g; Carbs: 43.4g; Fiber: 9.6g; Sugar: 26.6g

Choco Banana Smoothie

Servings: 1

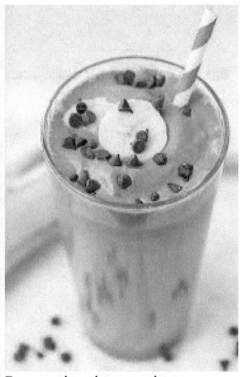

Preparation time: 5 minutes

Cooking time: 5 minutes

1 tsp maple syrup

1 tbsp cocoa powder

½ cup strawberries

1 banana

1 cup almond milk

Direction:

Add all ingredients into the blender and blend until smooth.

Serve and enjoy.

Nutrition: Calories: 709; Total Fat: 58.6g; Saturated Fat: 51.3g; Protein: 8.3g; Carbs: 53.2g; Fiber: 11.4g; Sugar: 30.1g

Tropical Smoothie

Servings: 1

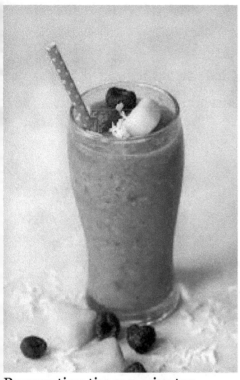

Preparation time: 5 minutes

Cooking time: 5 minutes

1 tsp collagen

1 tbsp coconut oil

6 oz pineapple juice

2/3 banana

4 strawberries

Direction:

Add all ingredients into the blender and blend until smooth.

Serve and enjoy.

Nutrition: Calories: 319; Total Fat: 14.2g; Saturated Fat: 11.9g; Protein: 7.8g; Carbs: 43.6g; Fiber: 3.4g; Sugar: 29g

Blueberry Smoothie

Servings: 1

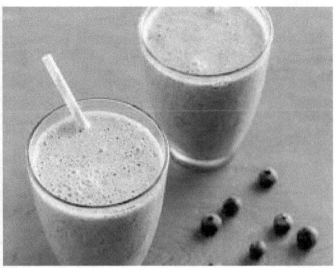

Preparation time: 5 minutes

Cooking time: 5 minutes

½ cup spinach

10 blueberries

1/3 banana

½ cup unsweetened almond milk

¼ cup ice cubes

2 tbsp chia seeds

Direction:

Add all ingredients into the blender and blend until smooth.

Serve and enjoy.

Nutrition: Calories: 517; Total Fat: 8.9g; Saturated Fat: 0.7g; Protein: 9.6g; Carbs: 112g; Fiber: 18.3g; Sugar: 72.4g

Acai Breakfast Bowl

Servings: 1

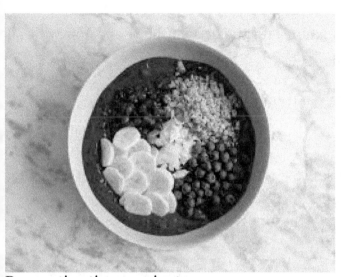

Preparation time: 5 minutes

Cooking time: 5 minutes

½ cup unsweetened almond milk

1 banana, frozen

2 tbsp acai powder

For toppings:

1 tsp flaxseeds

1 tsp almond butter

10 blueberries

3 strawberries, chopped

Direction:

Add acai powder, banana, and almond milk into the blender and blend until smooth.

Pour blended mixture into the serving bowl and top with all toppings ingredients.

Serve immediately and enjoy.

Nutrition: Calories: 636; Total Fat: 14.3g; Saturated Fat: 1.1g; Protein: 11g; Carbs: 132.9g; Fiber: 22.9g; Sugar: 84.5g

Chapter 7: Lunch

Asian Chicken and Rice Bowl

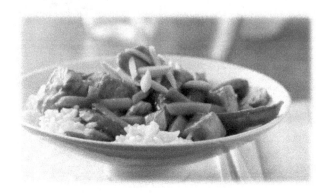

Servings: 4

Ingredients:

1 lb. boneless skinless chicken breast, sliced thin

1 ½ cups red bell pepper, sliced

6 cups fresh spinach, chopped

½ cup water chestnuts

1 tablespoon sesame oil

¼ cup soy sauce

1 tablespoon fresh grated ginger

½ teaspoon black pepper

½ cup peanuts, chopped

1 tablespoon sesame seeds

3 cups hot cooked basmati rice

Directions:

Heat the sesame oil in a skillet over medium to medium high heat.

Add the chicken and season it with the black pepper. Cook for 2 minutes.

Next, add in the red bell pepper and continue cooking for 2-3 minutes.

Add in the spinach, water chestnuts, and fresh grated ginger.

Sprinkle in the soy sauce and continue cooking until the spinach is wilted and the chicken is cooked through.

Serve the chicken and vegetable mixture over hot cooked basmati rice.

Garnish with sesame seeds and chopped peanuts before serving.

Nutrition: Calories: 534, Total Fat: 18.5g, Saturated Fat: 2.9g, Protein: 5.8g, Carbs: 10.8g, Fiber: 2.8g, Sugar: 5.9g

Brie Caprese Style Polenta

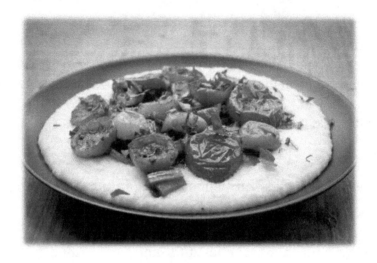

Servings: 4

Ingredients:

1 cup polenta

3 cups water or chicken broth

½ cup brie, cubed

1 tablespoon butter

½ teaspoon salt

½ teaspoon black pepper

1 tablespoon olive oil

1 medium tomato, sliced

½ cup fresh basil, chopped

Directions:

Preheat the oven to 350°F and line a baking sheet with aluminum foil.

Place the water or chicken broth in a large saucepan over medium heat.

Once the water warms, reduce the heat to medium low and stir in the polenta.

Continue cooking, stirring frequently to prevent sticking, for approximately 20 minutes, or until the polenta thickens.

While the polenta is cooking, place the tomato slices on the baking sheet and drizzle them with olive oil.

Place the baking sheet in the oven and bake for 10 minutes. Remove and set aside.

Season the polenta with the salt and black pepper. Add the butter and the brie and stir until the brie begins to melt into the polenta.

Transfer the polenta to serving dishes and top with the roasted tomato slices and fresh basil.

Nutrition: Calories: 127, Total Fat: 18.5g, Saturated Fat: 2.9g, Protein: 5g, Carbs: 10g, Fiber: 8g, Sugar: 9g

Salmon and Spinach

Preparation Time: 10 minutes

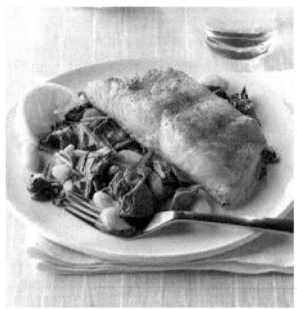

Cooking Time: 20 minutes

Servings: 4

Ingredients:

1 package gluten-free spaghetti noodles

1 tablespoon olive oil

1 ½ cup fresh spinach

1 can canned sliced mushrooms

2 cups lactose-free cream cheese

1 cup smoked salmon flakes

Juice from 1 lemon

Water

Salt and pepper to taste

Direction:

Place water in a deep pot and bring to a boil. Cook spaghetti noodles according to package Direction. Drain the noodles and set aside once cooked.

Heat olive oil in a pan over medium heat and wilt the spinach and set aside.

Using the same pan, stir in the mushrooms. Add in the cream cheese and pour water. Season with salt and pepper to taste. Bring to a boil and add in the salmon flakes.

Stir in the spaghetti noodles. Add the wilted spinach.

Drizzle with lemon juice before serving.

Nutrition: Calories 406, Total Fat 5.9 g, Saturated Fat 1.5g, Total Carbs 59.3g, Net Carbs 51g, Protein 32.5g, Sugar: 9.7g, Fiber: 8.3g, Sodium: 125mg, Potassium: 558mg

Spaghetti Bolognese

Preparation Time: 10 minutes

Cooking Time: 20 minutes

Servings: 5

Ingredients:

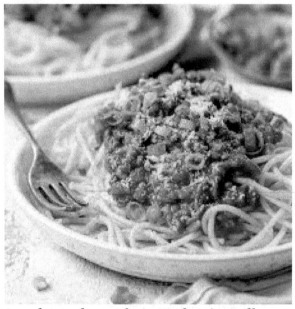

1 package gluten-free spaghetti noodles

1 tablespoon olive oil

½ lb. minced beef

1 cup green leeks, chopped

1 can crushed tomatoes

2 teaspoons Italian herbs

2 large carrots, grated

1 ½ cups chopped green beans

4 cups baby spinach, chopped

1 cup parmesan cheese

A handful of basil, torn

Salt and pepper to taste

Direction:

Cook the spaghetti noodles according to package Direction. Once cooked, drain the noodles and set aside.

Heat the olive oil over medium heat. Stir in the beef and leeks and cook for 3 minutes while stirring constantly.

Add in the tomatoes, herbs, carrots, and green beans. Season with salt and pepper to taste and adjust the moisture by adding more water if needed.

Allow to simmer for 10 minutes until the vegetables are soft.

Stir in the spinach and cooked noodles last.

Garnish with parmesan and basil leaves.

Nutrition: Calories 388, Total Fat 12.2g, Saturated Fat 4.4g, Total Carbs 49.9g, Net Carbs 40.2g, Protein 24.9g, Sugar: 4.6g, Fiber: 9.7g, Sodium: 491mg, Potassium: 652mg

Tuna Fried Rice

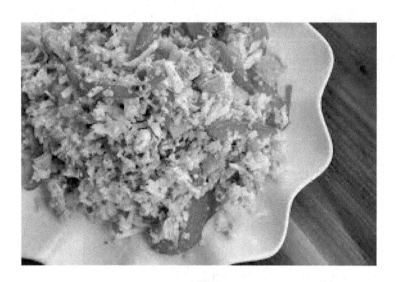

Preparation Time: 10 minutes

Cooking Time: 33 minutes

Servings: 4

Ingredients:

¼ tablespoon sesame oil

¼ tablespoon grated ginger

2 tablespoons green onions, green parts chopped

1/3 red bell pepper, seeded and sliced

1/3 carrot, peeled and grated

1 can tuna in brine, drained

1/3 cup long grain white rice

½ teaspoon Thai fish sauce

½ tablespoons soy sauce

2 tablespoons coriander leaves, chopped

Salt to taste

½ teaspoon white sugar

Direction:

Heat sesame oil in pan over medium flame. Sauté the ginger and green onions until fragrant.

Stir in the rest of the ingredients. Pour water to adjust the mixture. Give a good mix before covering the pan.

Cook on low for 30 minutes or until the rice is cooked through.

Nutrition: Calories 131, Total Fat 3.4g, Saturated Fat 0.9g, Total Carbs 13.7g, Net Carbs 13.2g, Protein 11.1g, Sugar: 0.9g, Fiber:0.5g, Sodium: 218mg, Potassium: 437mg.

Tuna Noodle Casserole

Preparation Time: 10 minutes

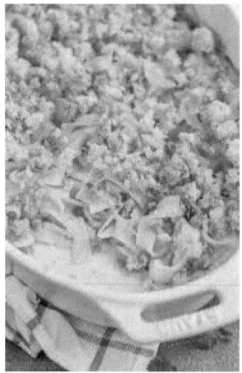

Cooking Time: 20 minutes

Servings: 4

Ingredients:

1 package 7 ounces gluten-free pasta

¼ cup unsalted butter

½ cup green part of the leek, chopped

½ cup green scallions, green part chopped

3 ½ ounces oyster mushrooms

¼ cup peas

¼ cup tapioca starch

¾ cup coconut milk

2 teaspoons soy sauce

2 ounces mozzarella cheese

Salt and pepper to taste

Direction:

Preheat the oven to 3500F. Grease the casserole dish with non-stick spray.

Cook the pasta in a large pot with boiling water and cook according to package Direction. Drain and set aside.

Melt the butter over medium heat in a skillet and sauté the leeks and scallion for 30 seconds. Stir in the oyster mushrooms and peas and cook for 2 minutes.

Stir in the tapioca starch and coconut milk. Allow to simmer and season with soy sauce, salt and pepper to taste.

Place the cooked pasta in the casserole dish and pour in the sauce.

Top with cheese.

Bake in the oven for 15 minutes.

Nutrition: Calories 262, Total Fat 19.1g, Saturated Fat 14.4g, Total Carbs 17.7g, Net Carbs 15g, Protein 7.5g, Sugar: 3.3g, Fiber: 2.7g, Sodium: 205mg, Potassium 290 mg

Italian Rice Bowl

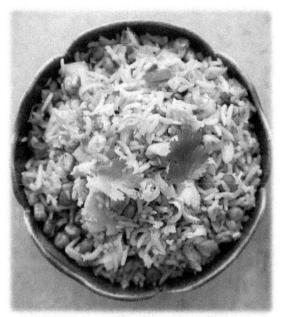

Ingredients:

1 tablespoon olive oil

1 cup long grain white rice

2 cups chicken broth (homemade or low-FODMAP)

½ teaspoon salt

½ teaspoon black pepper

¼ cup fresh basil, chopped

¼ fresh grated parmesan

½ lb. cooked, shredded chicken

2 cups radicchio, shredded or cut into strips

1 cup roasted red bell peppers

Directions:

Heat the olive oil in a skillet over medium heat.

Add the rice and cook while stirring until the rice is lightly toasted.

Add in the chicken broth, salt, and black pepper.

Increase the heat to medium high and bring the liquid to a boil.

Reduce the heat to low, cover and simmer for 20 minutes, or until the liquid is absorbed

Meanwhile, add a little more olive oil in a separate skillet.

Add in the radicchio and sauté for 5-7 minutes, or until it becomes tender. Add in the roasted red peppers and the chicken. Continue cooking, until warmed through.

Remove the lid from the rice and stir in the basil and the parmesan.

Transfer the rice to serving bowls and top with the chicken and vegetable mixture.

Nutrition: Calories 262, Total Fat 19.1g, Saturated Fat 14.4g, Total Carbs 17.7g, Net Carbs 15g, Protein 7.5g, Sugar: 3.3g, Fiber: 2.7g, Sodium: 205mg, Potassium 290 mg

Pineapple Chicken Skewers

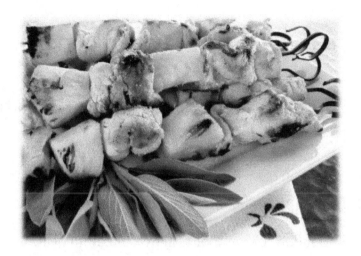

Servings: 4

Ingredients:

1 lb. boneless skinless chicken tenders, cut into cubes

¼ cup soy sauce

1 tablespoon brown sugar

2 teaspoons lime juice

2 teaspoons fresh grated ginger

1 cup fresh pineapple chunks

1 cup green bell pepper, cut into chunks

1 cup tomato, cut into chunks

Metal or bamboo skewers

Directions:

Begin by combining the soy sauce, brown sugar, lime juice and ginger in a bowl.

Add the chicken and let marinate for 30 minutes or longer in the refrigerator.

Meanwhile, if you are using bamboo skewers, soak them in water for at least 15 minutes before using to prevent burning.

Preheat and indoor or outdoor grill over medium heat.

Using an alternating pattern, place pieces of the chicken, pineapple, bell pepper and tomato on each skewer, making sure to leave a little bit of room between each addition to ensure even cooking.

Place the skewers on the grill and cook for 5-6 minutes per side, depending on the size of the chicken pieces, or until the chicken is cooked through.

Nutrition: Calories 262, Total Fat 19.1g, Saturated Fat 14.4g, Total Carbs 17.7g, Net Carbs 15g, Protein 7.5g, Sugar: 3.3g, Fiber: 2.7g, Sodium: 205mg, Potassium 290 mg

Chapter 8: Soups

Gingered Carrot Soup

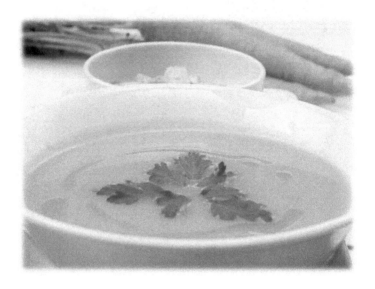

Servings: 4-6

Ingredients:

2 tablespoons butter

1 lb. carrots, peeled and diced

2 tablespoons fresh grated ginger

½ teaspoon salt

½ teaspoon black pepper

½ teaspoon cinnamon

½ teaspoon nutmeg

4 cups chicken or vegetable broth (FODMAP compliant)

1 cup cooked pumpkin, mashed

1 cup almond milk, or other FODMAP compliant milk alternative

¼ cup walnuts, chopped

¼ cup fresh parsley, chopped

Directions:

Add the butter to a large soup pan or stockpot.

Once the butter is hot, add in the carrots, salt, black pepper, cinnamon and nutmeg and sauté, stirring occasionally for 5-7 minutes or until tender.

Add the ginger and cook 1-2 additional minutes

Add in the broth, and increase the heat to medium high.

Bring the broth to a boil, then reduce the heat to low and simmer for 15 minutes.

Add the pumpkin to the soup, and using an immersion blender, blend until creamy. If you do not have an immersion blender, transfer the soup in batches to a traditional blender and puree until creamy.

Stir in the almond milk until desired consistency is reached.

Continue cooking over low heat for 5 minutes.

Serve garnished with fresh parsley and walnuts.

Nutrition: 253 calories, 121.8 mg calcium, 10.2 g fat, 2 mg iron, 2 g saturates, 16 g sugars, 0.4 g salt, 10.4 g protein, 1.5 g fiber and 48 g carbohydrates.

Rustic Potato Soup

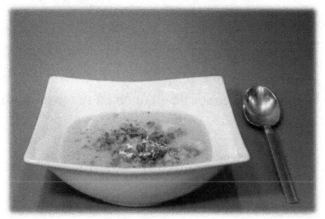

Servings: 6

Ingredients:

¼ lb. bacon, diced

6 medium sized potatoes, cut into cubes

2 cups carrots, diced

3 cups swiss chard, chopped

½ teaspoon salt

½ teaspoon black pepper

1 teaspoon dried thyme

¼ cup fresh parsley

2 tablespoons fresh chives

5 cups chicken or vegetable broth (FODMAP compliant)

½ cup fresh grated parmesan cheese

½ cup almond milk, or preferred FODMAP compliant milk alternative

Directions:

Place the bacon in a large soup pan or stock pot over medium high heat.

Cook the bacon, stirring frequently, until the bacon is browned and crisp.

Add the carrots, and cook while stirring for an additional 4-5 minutes.

Next, add in the swiss chard, potatoes, salt, black pepper, and thyme. Cook for 1-2 minutes.

Add in the broth and bring the liquid to a boil.

Once boiling, reduce the heat to low and simmer for 20 minutes, or until the potatoes and the carrots are tender.

Remove half of the soup, working in batches if necessary, and transfer it to a blender. Blend until creamy and then transfer it back into the pot with the rest of the soup.

Stir in the parsley, chives, parmesan cheese and almond milk.

Continue cooking over low heat for 5-10 minutes before serving.

Nutrition: 167 calories, 18 mg calcium, 10.2 g fat, 2.7 mg iron, 7 g saturates, 6 g sugars, 0.4 g salt, 14 g protein, 1.5 g fiber and 48 g carbohydrates.

Lemon Ginger Chicken and Rice Soup

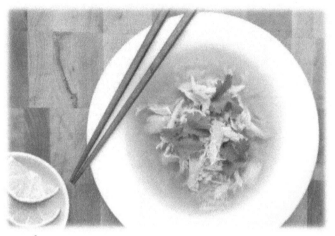

Servings: 4-6

Ingredients:

1 tablespoon olive oil

4 cups bok choy, shredded

2 tablespoons fresh grated ginger

1 teaspoon lemon zest

2 tablespoons soy sauce

2 tablespoons lemon juice

4-5 cups chicken broth (FODMAP compliant)

2 cups cooked, shredded chicken

2 cups cooked basmati rice

1 tablespoon fresh chives

Directions:

Heat the olive oil in a large soup pan or stock pot.

Once the oil is hot, add the bok choy, ginger and lemon zest. Cook, stirring frequently for 3-4 minutes.

Next, add in the lemon juice, soy sauce and chicken broth. Increase the heat to medium high and bring the liquid to a low boil.

Add in the shredded chicken and cooked rice. Reduce the heat to low and simmer for 10 minutes.

Serve garnished with fresh chives.

Nutrition: 323 calories, 121.8 mg calcium, 10.2 g fat, 2.7 mg iron, 2.2 g saturates, 19.6 g sugars, 0.4 g salt, 10.4 g protein, 1.5 g fiber and 46.8 g carbohydrates.

Ginger Carrot Soup

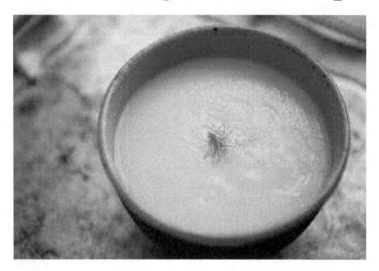

Preparation Time: 10 minutes

Cooking time: 20 minutes

Servings: 4

Ingredients:

12 carrots, peeled and diced

14 oz can coconut milk

2 cups vegetable broth, Low FODMAP

½ tsp cinnamon

2 fresh rosemary sprigs

1 Tbsp. fresh ginger, chopped

1 ½ tsp turmeric powder

2 Tbsp. olive oil

¼ tsp pepper

¼ tsp salt

Direction:

Preheat the oven to 400°F.

Place carrots on baking tray and drizzle with olive oil.

Roast carrots in preheated oven for 20 minutes.

Transfer roasted carrots in a food processor along with remaining ingredient and process until smooth.

Serve and enjoy.

Nutrition: Calories: 358, Total Fat: 29g, Saturated Fat: 20g, Protein: 6.1g, Carbs: 23.1g, Fiber: 5g, Sugar: 9.4g

Coconut Zucchini Soup

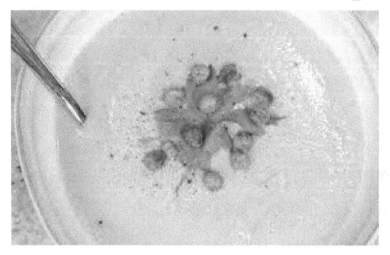

Preparation Time: 10 minutes

Cooking Time: 28 minutes

Servings: 4

Ingredients:

1 zucchini, chopped

1 bell pepper, chopped

2 carrots, chopped

1 cup of coconut milk

1 cup of water

1 Tbsp. olive oil

Direction:

Heat olive oil in a pan over medium heat.

Add vegetables to the pan and cook for 7-8 minutes or until they are done.

Add coconut milk and stir well, cook over medium heat for 5 minutes.

Add water and cook on low for 15 minutes.

Puree the soup using an immersion blender until smooth.

Season soup with pepper and salt.

Serve and enjoy.

Nutrition: Calories: 202, Total Fat: 18g, Saturated Fat: 13.2g, Protein: 2.8g, Carbs: 10.8g, Fiber: 3g, Sugar: 5.9g

Chicken Noodle Soup

Ingredients:

2-3 cup of chicken broth

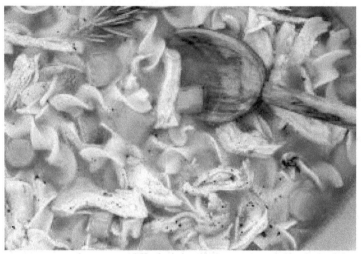

2-3 cups of water (fill the container used for broth)

1 cup of cooked, chopped chicken breast

2-4 oz. of uncooked gluten-free pasta/noodles

Salt and pepper to paste

Directions:

Add FODMAP Chicken Broth & Water into pot.

Bring to boil, stirring frequently.

Add Uncooked Gluten-Free Pasta & Chicken to pot.

Reduce heat & simmer for around 10 to12 minutes, stirring sporadically.

Add Salt and Pepper to taste, if desired.

When pasta is cooked to preference, remove from heat.

Serve immediately.

Makes about four servings.

Tomato Carrot Soup

Preparation Time: 10 minutes

Cooking Time: 4 hours Servings: 4

Ingredients:

4 medium carrots, peeled and chopped

1 tsp ground cumin

1 tsp ground coriander

1 Tbsp. turmeric

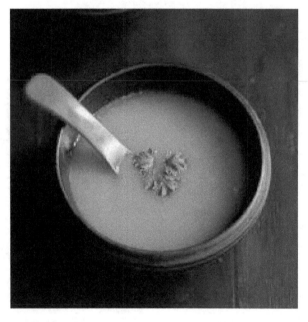

1 cup of coconut milk

14.5 oz can tomato, diced

Direction:

Add all Ingredients into the slow cooker and stir well.

Cover slow cooker with lid and cook on low for 4 hours.

Puree the soup using an immersion blender until smooth.

Serve and enjoy.

Nutrition: Calories: 193, Total Fat: 14.6g, Saturated Fat: 12.7g, Protein: 3g, Carbs: 15.9g, Fiber: 5g, Sugar: 8.6g

Tomato Basil Soup

Preparation Time: 10 minutes

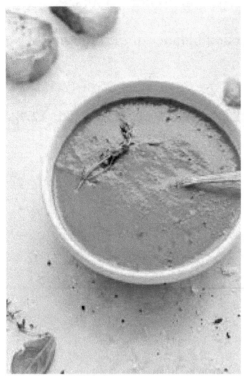

Cooking Time: 30 minutes

Servings: 4

Ingredients:

14 oz tomato, diced

2 tsp coriander

½ cup fresh basil, chopped

½ cup chicken broth, Low FODMAP

21 oz tomato puree

2 ½ cups fennel bulbs, chopped

1 ½ Tbsp. butter

Pepper

Salt

Direction:

Melt butter in a saucepan over medium heat.

Add fennel to the pan and sauté for 10 minutes over medium-high heat.

Add tomatoes, coriander, broth, and tomato puree and stir well. Bring to boil then turn heat to low and simmer for 20 minutes.

Remove from heat and stir in basil leaves.

Season the soup with pepper and salt.

Serve and enjoy.

Nutrition: Calories: 135, Total Fat: 5.1g, Saturated Fat: 2.9g, Protein: 4.8g, Carbs: 21.4g, Fiber: 5.8g, Sugar: 9.9g

Chapter 9: Salads

Dilly Egg Salad

Cooking Time: 10 minutes

Servings: 2

Ingredients:

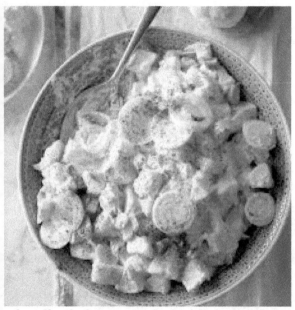

4 hardboiled eggs, peeled and chopped

1 tablespoon spicy mustard

½ teaspoon dill, dried

1 tablespoon mayonnaise

Salt and pepper

Direction:

Place all of the ingredients in a bowl. Mix well.

Season to taste.

Nutrition: 181 calories, 2 mg iron, 12.8 g fat, 81 mg calcium, 3.2 g saturates, 0.9-gram fiber, 12.6 g protein, 176 mg salts, 1.5 g sugars and 4.5 g carbohydrates.

Greek Chicken Salad

Cooking Time: 15 minutes

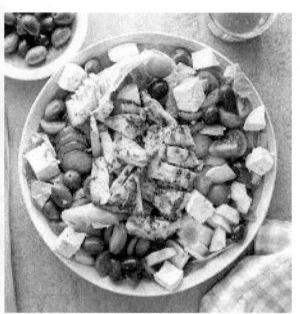

Servings: 6

Ingredients:

2 cups chicken, cooked and cubed

2 teaspoons lemon juice

1 plum tomato, diced

½ cup feta cheese, crumbled

1 tablespoon fresh oregano

¼ cup cucumber, peeled and diced

½ cup mayonnaise

12 olives, pitted

Salt and pepper

Direction:

Place chicken in a food processor. Blend until smooth.

Transfer chicken into a bowl. Add remaining ingredients and mix well. Season to taste.

Nutrition: 195 calories, 1 milligram iron, 11.7 g fat, 92 mg calcium, 3.4 g saturates, 0.8-gram fiber, 15.8 g protein, 0.4-gram salt, 2.2 g sugars and 6.8 g carbohydrates.

Dill and Cucumber Summer Salad

Cooking Time: 5 minutes

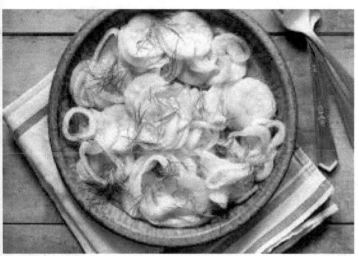

Servings: 1

Ingredients:

1 cucumber, halved and sliced

½ teaspoon lemon pepper

2 tablespoons fresh dill, chopped

Juice of 2 lemons

Direction:

Place all of the ingredients in a bowl and mix well.

Nutrition: 112 calories, 5 mg iron, 1.1-gram fat, 207 mg calcium, 7.3 g fiber, 0.2 gram saturates, 5.2 g protein, 23 mg salt, 9.2 g sugars and 30.7 g carbohydrates.

Egg and Potato Salad

Cooking Time: 25 minutes

Servings: 4

Ingredients:

800 g potato, cut into bite-sized pieces

1 tablespoon wholegrain mustard

160 g green beans, sliced

1 tablespoon lemon juice

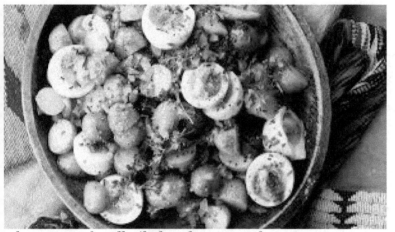

4 large eggs, hardboiled and quartered

3 tablespoons fresh chives, chopped

85 milliliters mayonnaise

1 red bell pepper

3 tablespoons green onions

1 small cucumber

Salt and pepper

Direction:

Place the potatoes in a large saucepan over medium high heat. Add enough amount of water to cover the potatoes.

Cover the saucepan with a lid and bring the water to a simmer. Reduce heat to medium low and allow to cook for 17 minutes.

Add green beans and cook for another 3 minutes. Once tender, drain the excess water and set the vegetables aside to cool.

Prepare the other vegetables. Peel off the skin of the cucumber and slice it into short sticks. Remove the white stem of the green onions and roughly chop the green tips. Dice the red bell peppers after removing the seeds.

Create the salad dressing by combining mustard, lemon juice and mayonnaise together. Season with black pepper to taste.

Place potatoes, green onions, cucumber, green beans, red bell pepper and eggs in a large bowl. Mix gently.

Drizzle with salad dressing and gently toss the salad.

Nutrition: 327 calories, 87.6 mg calcium, 11.2 g fat, 3.5 mg iron, 2.7 g saturates, 6.4 g sugars, 0.4 g salt, 13.5 g protein, 6.4 g fiber and 44.4 g carbohydrates.

Potato Salad

Preparation Time: 10 minutes

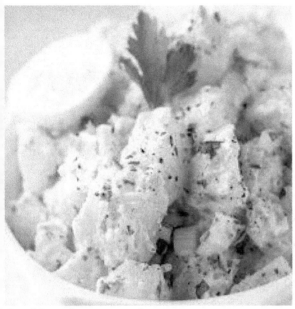

Cooking time: 20 minutes

Servings: 5

Ingredients:

1 lb. red potatoes

½ Tbsp. vinegar

1 Tbsp. Dijon mustard

½ lime zest

½ lime juice

2 Tbsp. olive oil

2 Tbsp. fresh dill, chopped

2 Tbsp. chives, minced

Pepper

Salt

Direction:

Add water in a large pot and bring to boil.

Add potatoes in boiling water and cook until tender, about 15 minutes. Drain well and set aside.

In a small bowl, whisk together vinegar, mustard, lime zest, lime juice, olive oil, dill, and chives.

Peel potatoes and diced. Place in mixing bowl.

Pour vinegar mixture over potatoes and stir until well coated.

Season with pepper and salt.

Serve and enjoy.

Nutrition: Calories: 148, Total Fat: 7.4g, Saturated Fat: 1.1g, Protein: 2.7g, Carbs: 19.7g; Fiber: 2.4g, Sugar: 1.3g

Fajita Salad

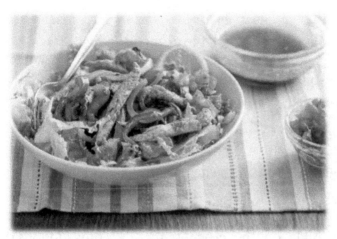

Servings: 4

Ingredients:

1 tablespoon olive oil

2 cups red bell peppers, sliced

2 cups zucchini, sliced

½ teaspoon salt

½ teaspoon black pepper

1 cup tomatoes, diced

6 cups baby spinach

¾ lb. cooked chicken, shredded and warmed

1 cup crushed tortilla chips (check ingredients for FODMAP approval)

Southwest Fajita Dressing

Directions:

Heat the olive oil in a skillet over medium heat.

Once the oil is hot, add in the red bell peppers and zucchini. Cooke the vegetables for approximately 5 minutes, or until the vegetables are firm tender.

Add the baby spinach to the serving plates and drizzle with the Southwest Fajita Dressing.

Next, sprinkle on the crushed tortilla chips, followed by the sautéed vegetables and chicken.

Nutrition: 327 calories, 121.8 mg calcium, 10.2 g fat, 2.7 mg iron, 2.2 g saturates, 19.6 g sugars, 0.4 g salt, 10.4 g protein, 1.5 g fiber and 46.8 g carbohydrates.

Quinoa Salad

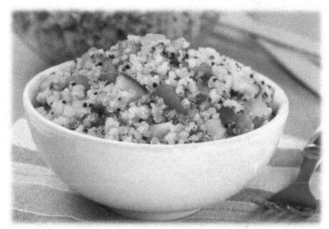

Servings: 4

Ingredients:

1 cup quinoa

2 cups water or FODMAP approved broth

3 tablespoons olive oil

1 ½ tablespoons lemon juice

¼ cup pine nuts

¾ cup roasted red peppers, chopped

1 cup kale, finely chopped

¾ cup feta cheese, crumbled

¼ cup fresh basil, chopped

½ teaspoon salt

½ teaspoon black pepper

Directions:

Combine the quinoa and water or broth in a saucepan over medium high heat.

Once the liquid comes to a boil, reduce the heat to low, cover and simmer for 15-20 minutes.

Remove the cover from the saucepan, fluff the quinoa and transfer it to a large bowl.

Whisk together the olive oil, lemon juice, salt and black pepper.

Drizzle the dressing over the quinoa and stir.

Add in the pine nuts, roasted red peppers, feta cheese and basil. Mix well.

Serve warm or cover and refrigerate until ready to serve.

Nutrition: Calories: 324; Total Fat: 40.3g; Saturated Fat: 26.5g; Protein: 11.6g; Carbs: 39.2g; Fiber: 9.4g; Sugar: 5.5g

Fruited Chicken Salad

Servings: 4

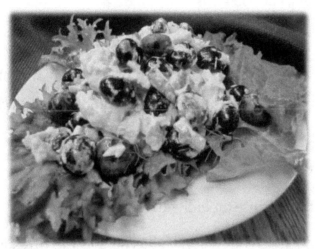

Ingredients:

6 cups baby spinach leaves

½ cup raspberries, halved

¾ cup blueberries

1 cup mandarin orange slices

3 tablespoons mayonnaise (check ingredients for FODMAP compliance)

2 tablespoons olive oil

1 teaspoon stone ground mustard

¼ cup feta cheese

2 tablespoons fresh mint

½ lb. cooked chicken, shredded or cubed

½ cup walnuts, chopped

Directions:

In a blender or food processor, combine the mayonnaise, olive oil, stone ground mustard, feta cheese, and mint. Blend until creamy.

In a bowl, spinach, raspberries, blueberries and mandarin orange slices. Toss to mix.

Place the salad mixture on individual serving plates.

In a separate bowl, combine the chicken and the dressing. Mix well.

Place equal sized portions of the dressed chicken on the salad.

Top with walnuts before serving.

Nutrition: Calories: 312; Total Fat: 43g; Saturated Fat: 25g; Protein: 11.6g; Carbs: 39.2g; Fiber: 9.4g; Sugar: 5.5g

Chef Salad

Servings: 4

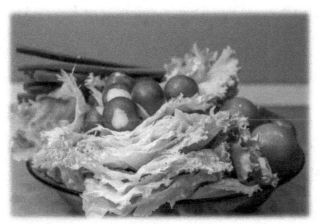

Ingredients:

6 cups butter lettuce, torn

1 ½ cups cooked turkey, cubed

2 eggs, hardboiled and halved

½ cup canned chickpeas, rinsed and drained

½ cup cucumber, sliced

½ cup radishes, sliced thin

¾ cup tomatoes, diced

¼ cup pumpkin seeds

Caper Dressing (see recipe)

Directions:

Divide the butter lettuce among the serving dishes.

Dress the salad greens with the caper dressing.

Arrange the turkey, chickpeas, cucumber, radishes and tomatoes on top of the salad in rows.

Garnish the salad with one half of a hardboiled egg and pumpkin seeds before serving.

Nutrition: Calories: 432; Total Fat: 40.3g; Saturated Fat: 26.5g; Protein: 16g; Carbs: 32g; Fiber: 9g; Sugar: 5g

Fruit and Protein Salad

Servings: 4

Ingredients:

6 cups baby spinach

2 cup cooked turkey, cubed or sliced

½ cup brussels sprouts, shaved

1 tablespoon olive oil

½ teaspoon salt

½ teaspoon black pepper

1 cup blueberries

½ cup feta cheese

½ cup walnuts

Raspberry Citrus Vinaigrette (see recipe)

Directions:

Heat the olive oil in a skillet over medium heat.

Once the oil is hot, add the brussels sprouts and season them with the salt and black pepper.

Sauté the shredded brussels sprouts for approximately 4-5 minutes, or until tender.

Remove the skillet from the heat and set aside.

In a bowl, combine the spinach, turkey, blueberries, and feta cheese.

Drizzle the salad Raspberry Citrus Vinaigrette over the salad and toss.

Transfer the salad to individual serving plates.

Top with the sautéed brussels sprouts and walnuts before serving.

Nutrition: Calories: 267; Total Fat: 46g; Saturated Fat: 25g; Protein: 11.6g; Carbs: 39.2g; Fiber: 9g; Sugar: 5g

Winter Roasted Vegetable Salad

Preparation Time: 5 minutes

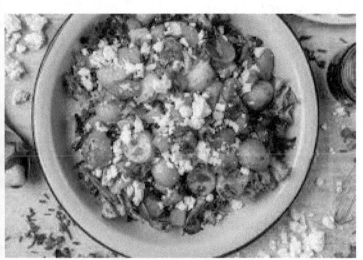

Cooking Time: 15 minutes

Servings: 2

Ingredients:

2 cups broccoli, cut into florets

2 cups yellow potatoes, scrubbed and halved

2 cups green beans

1 ½ teaspoon extra virgin olive oil

1 cup lettuce leaves

1 cup green onions, green part only

1 cup cooked quinoa

¼ cup red wine

¼ cup extra virgin olive oil

2 teaspoons Dijon mustard

Salt and pepper to taste

Direction:

Preheat the oven to 4000F.

Line a baking tray with parchment paper.

In a bowl, toss together the broccoli, potatoes, beans, and olive oil. Season with salt and pepper to taste.

Place seasoned vegetable in a baking tray.

Roast in the oven for 15 minutes. Make sure to toss the vegetables every 5 minutes for even cooking.

Place the roasted vegetables in a salad bowl and add in the lettuce, green onions and cooked quinoa.

Make the salad dressing by combining the red wine, olive oil, and mustard. Season with salt and pepper to taste.

Drizzle the dressing onto the salad.

Toss to coat.

Nutrition: Calories 408, Total Fat 16.3g, Saturated Fat 2.2g, Total Carbs 56.8g, Net Carbs 45.8g, Protein 11.1g, Sugar: 5.1g, Fiber: 11g, Sodium: 357mg, Potassium: 1167mg

Cobb Salad

Preparation Time: 10 minutes

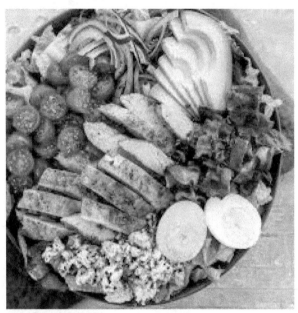

Cooking Time: 0 minutes

Servings: 4

Ingredients:

1 bag mixed salad greens, rinsed and chopped

2 big Roma tomatoes, diced

4 slices bacon, fried and crumbled

2 cups cooked chicken, shredded

4 hard-boiled eggs, diced

½ cup Kalamata olives, pitted and halved

¼ cup minced chives

2 tablespoons red wine vinegar

2 teaspoons Dijon mustard

1 teaspoon maple syrup

¼ cup olive oil

Salt and pepper to taste

Direction:

Place the salad greens, tomatoes, bacon, chicken, boiled eggs, olives, and chives in a bowl.

In another bowl, mix together the red wine vinegar, Dijon mustard, maple syrup, and olive oil Season with olive oil.

Drizzle the salad with the dressing and toss to coat.

Nutrition: Calories 645, Total Fat 58.1g, Saturated Fat 11g, Total Carbs 5.4g, Net Carbs 3.4g, Protein 24.6g, Sugar: 0.2g, Fiber: 2g, Sodium: 436mg, Potassium: 834mg

Fruit and Walnut Salad

Preparation Time: 5 minutes

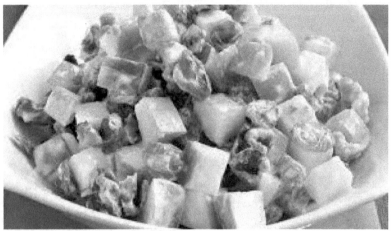

Cooking Time: 0 minutes

Servings: 1

Ingredients:

1 cup lettuce, torn

20 blueberries

1 tablespoon feta cheese, crumbled

10 walnut halves

Direction:

Dry the lettuce and place on a serving plate.

Crumble the feta cheese over the lettuce leaves and add fruits and nuts.

Nutrition: Calories 198, Total Fat 16.5g, Saturated Fat 3.3g, Total Carbs 9.2g, Net Carbs g, Protein 6.5g, Sugar: 4.9g, Fiber: 2.6g, Sodium: 252mg, Potassium: 277mg

Asian-Inspired Quinoa Salad

Preparation Time: 10 minutes

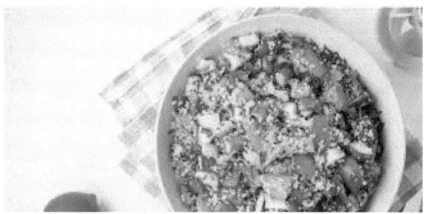

Cooking Time: 0 minutes

Servings: 4

Ingredients:

1 cup quinoa, cooked in 1 ½ cups of water

1 large red bell pepper, seeded and diced

2 medium Lebanese cucumbers, diced

1 large carrot, peeled and grated

½ cup fresh mint, chopped

½ cup coriander, chopped

Juice from 2 lemons

1 ½ tablespoons fish sauce

2 teaspoons minced ginger

2 teaspoons sesame oil

A dash of cayenne pepper

Salt and pepper to taste

Direction:

Place in a salad bowl the quinoa, red bell pepper, cucumber, carrots, mint, and coriander.

In another bowl, mix together the lemon juice, fish sauce, ginger, oil, and cayenne pepper. Season with salt and pepper to taste.

Drizzle the dressing over the salad and toss to coat.

Nutrition: Calories 153, Total Fat 6g, Saturated Fat 1.5g, Total Carbs 17.8g, Net Carbs 14.7g, Protein 8.7g, Sugar: 4.7g, Fiber: 3.1g, Sodium: 775mg, Potassium: 472mg

Low FODMAP Potato Salad

Preparation Time: 5 minutes

Cooking Time: 10 minutes

Servings: 2

Ingredients:

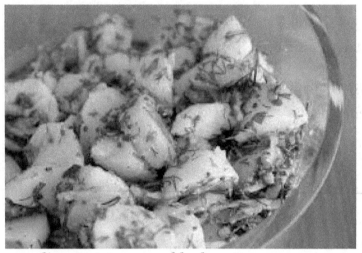

4 medium potatoes, scrubbed

5 slices of bacon

2 drops balsamic vinegar

2 drops olive oil

Fresh mint for garnish, chopped

Salt and pepper to taste

Direction:

Boil the potatoes in a pot for 10 minutes or until soft. Drain and peel.

Meanwhile, fry the bacon for 3 minutes on each side or until crispy. Crumble.

Slice the potatoes and place in a bowl. Season with balsamic vinegar, olive oil, salt and pepper to taste.

Garnish with mint last.

Nutrition: Calories 833, Total Fat 26.2g, Saturated Fat 0.1g, Total Carbs 74.9g, Net Carbs 65.6g, Protein 16.7g, Sugar: 3.8g, Fiber: 9.4g, Sodium: 331mg, Potassium: 674mg

Egg and Bacon Salad

Cooking Time: 15 minutes

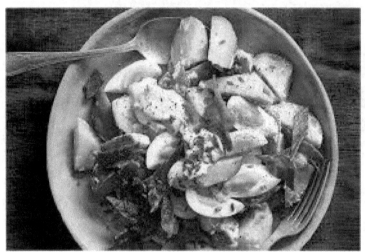

Servings: 2

Ingredients:

2 large hardboiled eggs, quartered

2 medium tomatoes, cut into small pieces

100 g bacon strips

1 small cucumber, peeled and sliced

30 g baby spinach

1 teaspoon garlic-infused oil

4 tablespoons mayonnaise

Salt and pepper

Direction:

Over medium heat, fry the bacon strips in a pan for about 5 minutes or until crispy. Slice the bacon into smaller pieces.

Mix oil and mayonnaise together until well combined. Season with black pepper to taste.

Spread the mayonnaise mixture at the bottom of a mason jar. Arrange layers of tomatoes, cucumber, spinach, eggs and bacon on top.

Store the salad in the refrigerator.

Nutrition: 429 calories, 82 mg calcium, 35 g fat, 2.4 mg iron, 10 g saturates, 7 g sugars, 0.7 g salt, 16.5 g protein, 2.6 g fiber and 13 g carbohydrates.

Summer Beef Salad

Cooking Time: 15 minutes

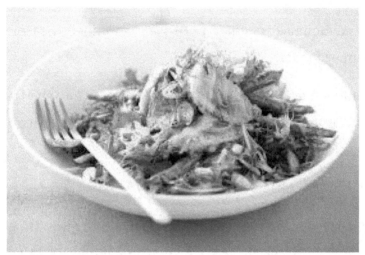

Servings: 4

Ingredients:

600 g beef rump steak

10 g green onions

1 tablespoon canola oil

16 pieces cherry tomatoes

180 g green beans, trimmed and sliced

1 red bell pepper

6 cups red coral lettuce, shredded

1 ½ tablespoon Dijon mustard

¼ teaspoon white sugar

2 tablespoons white vinegar

¼ teaspoon black pepper

60 milliliters olive oil

Direction:

Slice the red bell pepper into strips after removing the seeds. Remove the white stem of the green onions and slice the green tips finely. Cut the tomatoes in half.

Grill the red bell pepper strips in the oven at 220 degrees Celsius. Once the skin turned black, remove the bell pepper from the oven.

Allow the bell pepper to cool before removing the blackened skin.

Rub each side of the side with oil and season to taste. In a large frying pan, cook the steak to your liking over medium-high heat. Slice the meat thinly after letting it rest for about 5 minutes.

Place the green beans in boiling water. Rinse the beans under cold water after blanching it for 2 minutes and drain any excess water.

Make a mustard vinaigrette by combining white vinegar, sugar, Dijon mustard and olive oil together. Stir well and season with black pepper to taste.

Place green beans, red bell pepper, lettuce and cherry tomatoes on a bowl and mix well. Place steak slices on top and drizzle with mustard vinaigrette.

Nutrition: 436 calories, 57.8 mg calcium, 27.6 g fat, 5 mg iron, 6.8 g saturates, 8.4 g sugars, 0.3 g salt, 36.5 g protein, 3.7 g fiber and 13.2 g carbohydrates.

Rosemary Chicken Salad

Preparation Time: 5 minutes

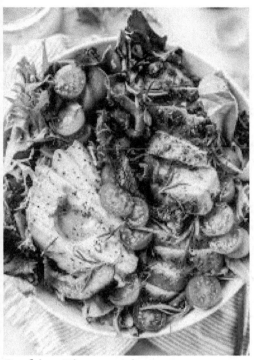

Cooking Time: 7 minutes

Servings: 5

Ingredients:

3 cups grilled chicken, cubed

2 Tbsps. plain yogurt, lactose-free

¼ cup sliced toasted almonds

½ cup mayonnaise, full-fat

1 Tbsp. red wine vinegar

1 tsp crumbled dried rosemary

3 cups seedless grapes, sliced

Direction:

For dressing: Whisk together rosemary, vinegar, yogurt, and mayonnaise in a small bowl.

Combine chicken with grapes and dressing in a large bowl and toss to combine.

Use almonds to and then serve.

Nutrition: Calories: 320 , Fat: 17g , Protein: 26g , Sodium: 210mg , Fiber: 1g , Carbohydrates: 16g , Sugar: 12g

Summer Salad

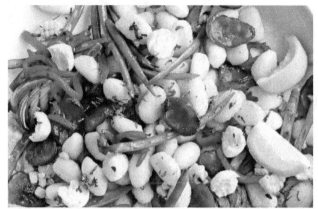

Preparation Time: 10 minutes

Cooking Time: 5 minutes

Servings: 2

Ingredients:

2 cups lettuce

2 Tbsp. feta cheese, crumbled

¼ cup walnuts, chopped

1/3 cup strawberries, sliced

½ cup blueberries

For dressing:

1 Tbsp. apple cider vinegar

1 Tbsp. olive oil

Pepper

Salt

Direction:

In a medium bowl, mix together lettuce, strawberries, blueberries, and walnuts.

In a small bowl, whisk together all dressing Ingredients.

Pour dressing over salad and mix well.

Top with crumbled cheese and serve.

Nutrition: Calories: 219, Total Fat: 18.5g, Saturated Fat: 2.9g, Protein: 5.8g, Carbs: 10.8g, Fiber: 2.8g, Sugar: 5.9g

Refreshing Cucumber Tomato Salad

Preparation Time: 15 minutes

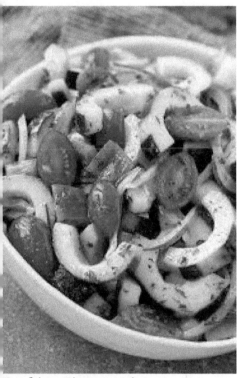

Cooking Time: 5 minutes

Servings: 8

Ingredients:

1 large cucumber, diced

2 Tbsp. fresh dill, chopped

½ cup feta cheese, crumbled

½ cup olives, drained and chopped

16 cherry tomatoes, quartered

For dressing:

1 tsp dried oregano

1 Tbsp. fresh dill, minced

1 tsp sugar

¼ cup rice wine vinegar

1/3 cup olive oil

Pepper

Salt

Direction:

Add all salad Ingredients into the mixing bowl and mix well.

In a small bowl, whisk together all dressing Ingredients.

Pour dressing over salad and toss well.

Serve and enjoy.

Nutrition: Calories: 167, Total Fat: 11.9g, Saturated Fat: 2.8g, Protein: 4.1g, Carbs: 13.1g, Fiber: 3.7g, Sugar: 8g

Moroccan Chicken Salad

Cooking Time: 10 minutes

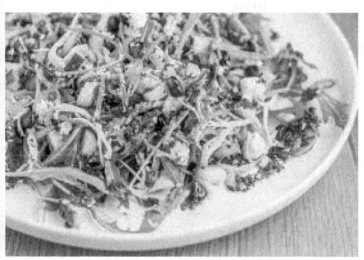

Servings: 2

Ingredients:

250 g skinless chicken breast, cubed

1/8 teaspoon white sugar

½ tablespoon garlic-infused oil

1/8 teaspoon ginger, ground

¼ teaspoon cumin, ground

½ teaspoon paprika

1/8 teaspoon turmeric, ground

¼ teaspoon coriander, ground

2 tablespoons olive oil

½ tablespoon pure maple syrup

1 tablespoon fresh orange juice

1 small cucumber

60 g lettuce leaves, assorted

1 red bell pepper, diced and deseeded

2 imperial mandarin, peeled

Salt and pepper

Direction:

Place oil, sugar, cumin, ginger, coriander, turmeric and paprika in a bowl. Coat chicken cubes with the spice mixture. Season with salt and pepper to taste.

Stir-fry chicken over medium-high heat for about 4 minutes. Set aside to cool.

Combine orange juice, olive oil, ¼ teaspoon salt and maple syrup together to create orange dressing. Season with black pepper.

Mix all of the ingredients in a bowl.

Nutrition: 398 calories, 67.6 mg calcium, 21.5 g fat, 1.9 mg iron, 3.2 g saturates, 14.6 g sugars, 0.5 g salt, 30.6 g protein, 4 g fiber and 21.3 g carbohydrates.

Chapter 10: Dinner

Gluten-free Chicken & Vegetable Pie

Ingredients:

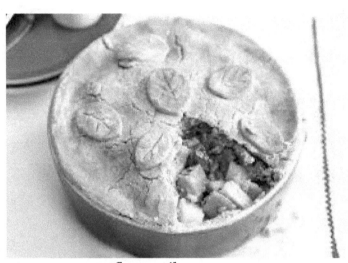

1 teaspoons sunflower oil

1 garlic of clove, finely chopped

400 g chicken breast fillet, diced

1 med. zucchini, chopped

1 med. carrot, peeled, chopped

1 med. potato, peeled & diced

2 cups gluten-free chicken stock

2 tbsp. gluten-free corn flour

1/4 cup chopped/fresh flat-leaf parsley leaves

1/4 cup fresh tarragon leaves - finely chopped

1 pie pastry (see related recipe)

1 egg - lightly beaten

Direction:

Preheat oven to 200°C/180°C fan forced. Heat oil in saucepan over med. heat. Add garlic & chicken. Cook - stirring for 5 minutes or until nicely browned. Add zucchini, carrots and potato. Cook for three minutes. Add one cup of stock to pan.

Place corn flour and 1/4 cup remaining stock in bowl. Stir in order to form a paste. Stir in remaining stock. Stir corn flour mixture into chicken mixture. Bring to boil. Reduce heat to medium-low. Simmer for five minutes or until thickened. Stir in parsley & tarragon. Spoon mixture into a five-cup capacity ovenproof dish.

Make pastry: roll pastry out on a lightly floured surface until big enough to cover a dish. Place pastry over filling. Pinch the edges to seal. Brush with egg. Bake for 35-40 minutes or until pastry is golden brown. Let stand for five minutes to cool. Serve.

Nutritional Information:

Energy 1652 kJ

Fat Saturated 3.60 g

Fat Total 20.90 g

Carbohydrate Total 30.80 g

Dietary Fiber 2.30 g

Protein 19.30 g

Cholesterol 75.00 mg

Sodium 622.00 mg

Pad Thai With Shrimps

Preparation Time: 10 minutes

Cooking Time: 6 minutes

Servings: 4

Ingredients:

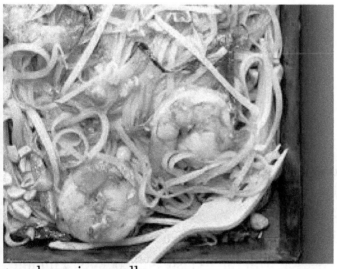

1 package rice noodle

2 tablespoons olive oil

1 lb. large shrimps, peeled and deveined

1 red bell pepper, thinly sliced

¼ cup fish sauce

¼ cup white sugar

2 tablespoons rice vinegar

1 tablespoons ground paprika

2 teaspoons low sodium tamari

1 large egg, fried and cut into strips

2 green onions, green parts only chopped

1 cup fresh bean sprouts

1 teaspoon sesame seeds

Freshly chopped cilantro leaves

Salt to taste

Direction:

Cook the rice noodles according to package Direction. Drain and set aside.

Heat the olive oil in pan over medium heat and stir in the shrimps and bell pepper. Season with salt to taste and cook for 4 minutes until the shrimps turn red. Set aside.

In a mixing bowl, combine the fish sauce, white sugar, rice vinegar, and paprika. Add in the tamari.

Assemble the Pad Thai. Place the noodles at the bottom of the bowl and place the shrimps and bell pepper on top. Add egg strips, green onions, and bean sprouts. Drizzle with the sauce.

Garnish with sesame seeds and cilantro seeds.

Nutrition: Calories 429, Total Fat 13.5g, Saturated Fat 2g, Total Carbs 52.7g, Net Carbs 48.5g, Protein 24.4g, Sugar: 4.7g, Fiber: 4.2g, Sodium: 215mg, Potassium: 423mg

Coconut Chicken Rice Noodle

Preparation Time: 5 minutes

Cooking Time: 10 minutes

Servings: 4

Ingredients:

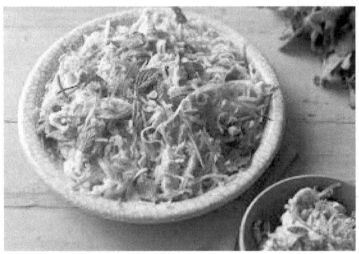

1 package rice noodle

2 tablespoons coconut oil

1 lb. chicken breasts

1 zucchini, sliced

1 bell pepper, seeded and sliced

2 carrots, peeled and sliced

1 can coconut milk

Salt and pepper to taste

Direction:

Cook the rice noodles according to package Direction. Drain and set aside.

Heat coconut oil in a deep pan over medium heat and fry the chicken breasts for 3 minutes on each side or until they turn golden brown.

Stir in the zucchini, bell pepper, and carrots. Season with salt and pepper to taste. Stir for 1 minute.

Add in the coconut milk.

Cover the pan with lid and simmer for 6 minutes.

Add cooked noodles last.

Nutrition: Calories 415, Total Fat 13.9g, Saturated Fat 7.1g, Total Carbs 22.5g, Net Carbs 19.1g, Protein 19.6g, Sugar: 1.2g, Fiber: 3.4g, Sodium: 102mg, Potassium: 347mg

Beef and Vegetable Stir Fry with Oyster Sauce

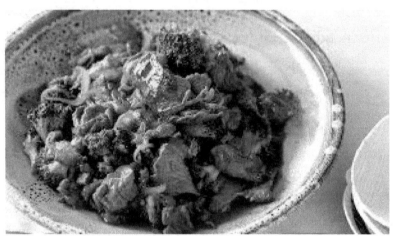

Preparation Time: 10 minutes

Cooking Time: 15 minutes

Servings: 2

Ingredients:

2 tablespoons sesame oil

½ lb. beef slices

½ carrot, peeled and julienned

½ cup broccoli florets

½ cup chopped bok choy

6 oz rice noodles

2 tablespoons oyster sauce

1 teaspoon lime juice

Salt and pepper to taste

Water

Direction:

Heat the sesame oil in pan over medium flame and stir in the beef slices. Season with salt and pepper to taste. Cook for 3 minutes.

Stir in the vegetables and rice noodles. Pour in a few tablespoons of water to adjust the moisture. Season with oyster sauce.

Keep stirring until the noodles and vegetables are cooked.

Drizzle with lime juice last.

Nutrition: Calories 611, Total Fat 49.5g, Saturated Fat 16.4g, Total Carbs 11.7g, Net Carbs 10.7g, Protein 29.7g, Sugar: 5.3g, Fiber: 1g, Sodium: 638mg, Potassium: 503mg

Chicken and Rice

Preparation Time: 5 minutes

Cooking Time: 35 minutes

Servings: 4

Ingredients:

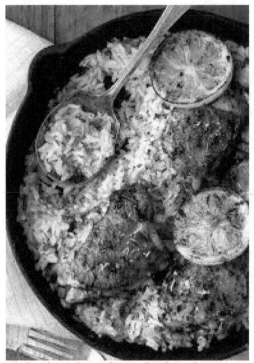

4 skinless boneless chicken breasts, around 1 ½ lbs.

1 ¾ teaspoon ground cumin

1 ¾ teaspoon paprika powder

1 tablespoon coconut oil

1 red and green bell peppers, seeded and chopped

1 large tomato, chopped

1 tablespoon ginger, chopped

1 teaspoon turmeric powder

1 cup white rice, uncooked

Salt and pepper to taste

2 cups water

Direction:

Season the chicken breasts with cumin, paprika, salt, and pepper.

Heat oil in a pan over medium flame and stir in the seasoned chicken breasts. Allow to brown on all sides for at least 3 to 4 minutes. Set aside.

Using the same pan, stir in the green bell peppers, tomatoes, ginger, and turmeric. Allow the vegetables to sweat.

Add the rice and season with salt and pepper to taste. Pour in water.

Put lid on the pan and cook the rice for 30 minutes on low heat.

Halfway through the cooking time, place the chicken on top of the rice and continue cooking.

Nutrition: Calories 545, Total Fat 11.2g, Saturated Fat 4.6g, Total Carbs 41.3g, Net Carbs 38.8g, Protein 65.2g, Sugar: 1.4g, Fiber: 2.5g, Sodium: 131mg, Potassium: 1113mg

Mediterranean Baked Fish

Ingredients:

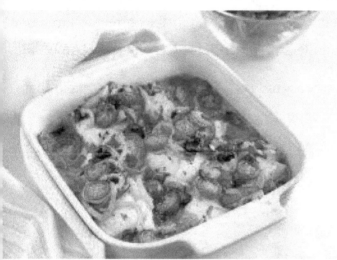

750 g. of baby new potatoes (cut larger potatoes into halves)

250 g. of cherry tomatoes, on the vine

70 g. of pitted black olives

4 skinless haddock fillets (or similar white fish)

2 tablespoons of garlic flavored olive oil

Juice of one lemon

A pinch of salt & pepper

A large handful of fresh basil leaves coarsely chopped or torn

Directions:

In a med. sauce pan, bring water to boil. Add quinoa & 1 teaspoon of salt & bring to boil. Reduce heat to low, cover & simmer until water is absorbed, 15-20 minutes. Transfer quinoa to large bowl & immediately add lemon juice, olive oil & one teaspoon of salt.

Gently fold in green onions – mint – parsley – cucumbers - tomatoes & black pepper.

Gently fold in Feta cheese & season with additional salt & pepper, if desired. Serve at room temperature or a little chilled.

Chapter 11: Smoothie Recipes

Strawberry Smoothie

Preparation Time: 2 minutes

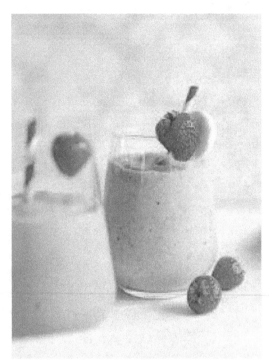

Cooking Time: 0 minutes

Servings: 1

Ingredients:

½ cup coconut milk

1 can fresh strawberries

¼ cup vanilla soy ice cream

1 ½ teaspoon rice protein powder

1 teaspoon chia seeds

½ tablespoon maple syrup

1 teaspoon lemon juice

6 ice cubes

Direction:

Place all ingredients in a blender.

Pulse until smooth.

Serve while still cold.

Nutrition: Calories 168, Total Fat 4.1g, Saturated Fat 0.5g, Total Carbs 21.4g, Net Carbs 15.4g, Protein 13.9g, Sugar: 11.2g, Fiber: 6g, Sodium: 75mg, Potassium: 353mg

Oatmeal Cookie Breakfast Smoothie

Preparation Time: 2 minutes

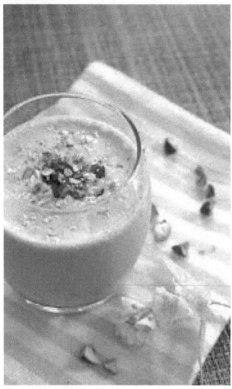

Cooking Time: 0 minutes

Servings: 1

Ingredients:

1 yellow banana, peeled and sliced

¾ cup almond milk

¼ cup ice

1/8 tablespoon vanilla

½ teaspoon cinnamon powder

2 tablespoons rolled oats

A dash of ground nutmeg

Direction:

Place all ingredients in a blender.

Pulse until smooth.

Serve immediately.

Nutrition: Calories 303, Total Fat 7.8g, Saturated Fat 2.5g, Total Carbs 60g, Net Carbs 52.1g, Protein 5.5g, Sugar: 32.6g, Fiber: 7.9g, Sodium: 146mg, Potassium: 698mg

Matcha and Kiwi Smoothie

Ingredients for 2 smoothies

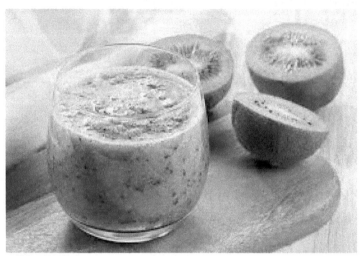

2 kiwi, ripe

1 teaspoons of matcha powder

1 banana, ripe

280 ml (1/4 cup) almond milk (unsweetened)

Direction: Snip the banana into small pieces, put it in a freezer bag and store it in the freezer for at least 3,5 hours (overnight would be perfect).

After this time, place all the ingredients in a powerful blender or food processor.

Blend until creamy.

Offer immediately.

Green Kiwi Smoothie

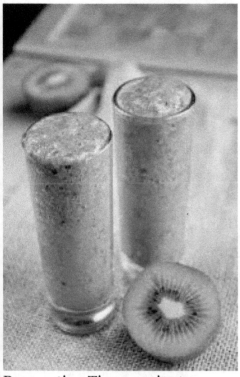

Preparation Time: 3 minutes

Cooking Time: 0 minutes

Servings: 2

Ingredients:

1 cup seedless green grapes

1 kiwi, peeled and chopped

2 tablespoons water

8 inches cucumber, cut into chunks

2 cups baby spinach

1 ½ cups ice cubes

1 green apple, peeled and cored

Direction:

Place all ingredients in a blender.

Pulse until the mixture becomes smooth.

Serve immediately.

Nutrition: Calories 132, Total Fat 1 g, Saturated Fat 0.5g, Total Carbs 33g, Net Carbs 30g, Protein 3g, Sugar: 25g, Fiber: 3g, Sodium: 4mg, Potassium: 226mg

Pumpkin Smoothie

Preparation Time: 2 minutes

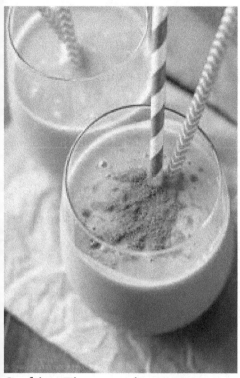

Cooking Time: 0 minutes

Servings: 1

Ingredients:

½ frozen medium ripe bananas, peeled and sliced

¼ cup pumpkin puree

½ cup coconut milk

¼ teaspoon pumpkin pie spice

1 tablespoon maple syrup

½ cup crushed ice

A pinch of cinnamon

Direction:

Place all ingredients in a blender except for the cinnamon.

Blend until smooth.

Put into glasses and sprinkle with cinnamon before serving.

Nutrition: Calories 695, Total Fat 37.7g, Saturated Fat 30g, Total Carbs 52.3g, Net Carbs 43.1g, Protein 14.3g, Sugar: 29.6g, Fiber: 9.2g, Sodium: 56mg, Potassium: 829mg

Chocolate Sesame Smoothie

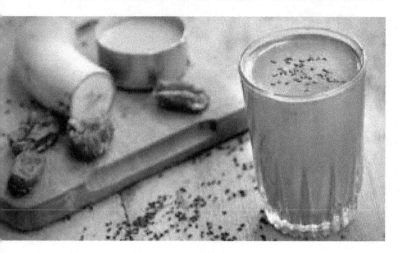

Preparation Time: 2 minutes

Cooking Time: 0 minutes

Servings: 1

Ingredients:

1 tablespoon sesame seeds

2 teaspoons unsweetened raw cocoa powder

Half of a medium banana, peeled and sliced

Flesh from 1/8 slice of avocado

1 tablespoon maple syrup

1 cup coconut milk

½ cup ice

Direction:

Place all ingredients in a blender.

Pulse until smooth.

Pour in a glass and serve immediately.

Nutrition: Calories 406, Total Fat 17.5g, Saturated Fat 6.3g, Total Carbs 57.3g, Net Carbs 50.5g, Protein 11.8g, Sugar: 39.2g, Fiber: 6.8g, Sodium: 115mg, Potassium: 1033mg

Chapter 12: Dessert and snacks

No-Bake Energy Bars

Cooking Time: 10 minutes

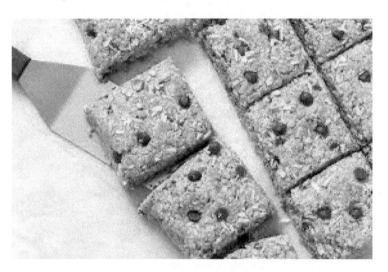

Servings: 14

Ingredients:

1/3 cup peanut butter

½ teaspoon guar gum

6 tablespoons pure maple syrup

15 g dark chocolate, chopped

45 g puffed rice

½ teaspoon cinnamon, ground

75 g pumpkin seeds, chopped

½ teaspoon ginger, ground

4 tablespoons cranberries, dried and chopped

Direction:

Place peanut butter and maple syrup in a frying pan. Melt peanut butter over medium heat and stir well.

Remove from heat. Except for chocolate, add all of the ingredients to the mixture and combine thoroughly.

Transfer the contents of the pan in a square pan lined with baking paper. Spread evenly.

Cover the mixture with another piece of baking paper. Press firmly.

Heat the chocolate in the microwave until melted. Stir every 30 minutes.

Drizzle melted chocolate over the energy bar mixture. Refrigerate for 10 minutes before cutting into bars.

Nutrition: 121 calories, 18.1 mg calcium, 6.4 g fat, 1.9 mg iron, 1 gram saturates, 1.2 g fiber, 3 g protein, 8.8 g sugars and 14.4 g carbohydrates.

Frozen Yogurt Bark with Berries

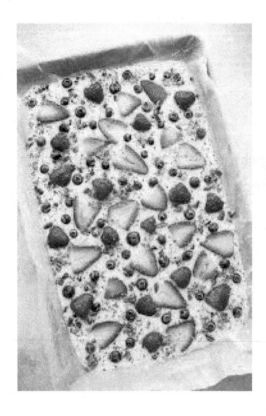

Cooking Time: 5 minutes

Servings: 10

Ingredients:

300 g coconut yogurt

8 pieces raspberries, crumbled

5 pieces fresh strawberries, chopped

2 tablespoons strawberry jam, melted

15 pieces fresh blueberries

1 teaspoon vanilla extract

Direction:

Combine yogurt and vanilla extract together.

Spread the mixture evenly in a square pan lined with baking paper. Ensure that it is thick enough to hold fruit bits.

Place a dollop of strawberry jam in the yogurt and stir roughly to create swirls. Distribute berries on top.

Left it in the freezer for about 3 hours before cutting.

Nutrition: 44 calories, 37.9 mg calcium, 0.4 g fat, 0.1 mg iron, 0.2 g saturates, 0.5 g fiber, 1.2 g protein, 6.6 g sugars and 8.4 g carbohydrates.

Coconut Macaroons

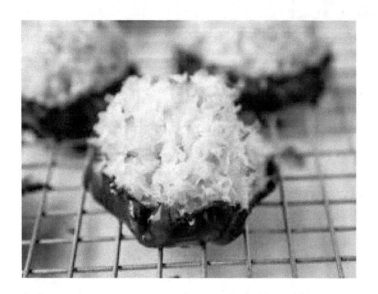

Cooking Time: 20 minutes

Servings: 24

Ingredients:

240 g coconut, dried and shredded

1/8 teaspoon salt

½ teaspoon lemon zest

4 egg whites

1 teaspoon vanilla extract

208 g white sugar

Direction:

Set the oven to 160 degrees Celsius.

Place the coconut in a roasting tray. Toast for about 5 minutes. Toss the coconut twice throughout the cook. Set aside to cool.

Whisk the remaining ingredients together until frothy.

Add coconut into the mixture and mix gently.

Create 3-cm coconut balls and place them in a roasting tray lined with baking paper. Make sure to leave enough space in between the balls.

Bake the macaroons for about 20 minutes. Once golden, set aside to cool for 5 minutes.

Nutrition: 103 calories, 3.2 mg calcium, 6.5 g fat, 0.3 mg iron, 5.7 g saturates, 1.6 g fiber, 1.3 g protein 9.5 g sugars and 11.1 g carbohydrates.

Curried Chickpea and Carrot Frittata

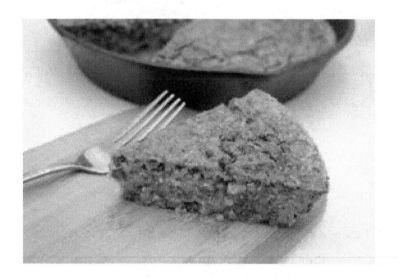

Cooking Time: 30 minutes

Servings: 16

Ingredients:

320 g carrot, peeled and diced

168 g canned chickpeas, rinsed and drained

4 large eggs

5 tablespoons fresh cilantro, chopped

313 milliliters almond milk

116 g firm tofu, drained and chopped

50 g butter, melted

1 ½ teaspoon mild curry powder

240 g zucchini, grated

2 teaspoons garlic-infused oil

40 g green onions

105 g self-rising flour, gluten-free

Salt and pepper

Direction:

Set the oven to 180 degrees Celsius.

Saute carrots in olive oil for about 15 minutes while stirring occasionally.

Combine eggs, oil, butter and milk together in a large bowl. Add flour and curry powder. Mix well.

Remove the white stems of the green onions and chop the green tips finely. Add the green onion tips to the egg mixture together with zucchini, carrots, chickpeas, cilantro and tofu. Season to taste and stir well.

Pour the mixture into a muffin tray lined with paper cups. Bake for 30 minutes.

Nutrition: 118 calories, 67.9 mg calcium, 5.5 g fat, 0.9 mg iron, 1 gram saturates, 3.1 g sugars, 0.1-gram salt, 4.4 g protein, 1.7 g fiber and 12.4 g carbohydrates.

Yummy Brownie Balls

Preparation Time: 50 minutes

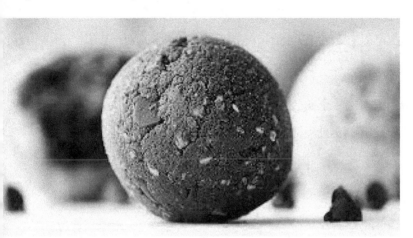

Servings: 20

Ingredients:

2 Tbsp. chia seeds

2 Tbsp. unsweetened cocoa powder

¼ cup maple syrup

3 Tbsp. chocolate chips

½ cup unsweetened peanut butter

1 cup rolled oats, gluten-free

Direction:

Add peanut butter and oats into the food processor and process until oats are just mixed with butter.

Now add remaining Ingredients and process until just mixed.

Make small balls from mixture and place on a parchment-lined dish.

Once done, place in refrigerator until brownie balls no longer sticky.

Nutrition: Calories: 75, Total Fat: 4. 3g, Saturated Fat: 1g, Protein: 2.1g, Carbs: 8g, Fiber: 1g, Sugar: 3.6g

Berry Crumb Cake

Preparation Time: 20 minutes

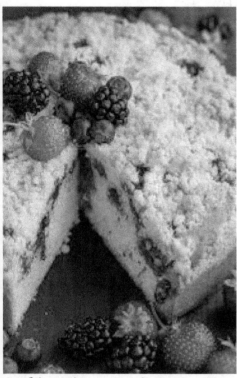

Cooking Time: 50 minutes

Servings: 16

Ingredients:

2 cups gluten-free flour

1 teaspoon baking powder

¾ cup butter, cold

¾ cup coconut milk

1 tablespoon lemon juice

2 eggs

1 cup strawberries and blueberries

1 cup sugar

Direction:

Preheat the oven to 3500F and lightly grease an 8x8 square pan.

In a bowl, add the sugar, baking powder, and sugar.

Add butter into the flour mixture gradually. Use a pastry blender until you achieve a crumb-like texture. Reserve half of the crumb mixture for the topping.

In another bowl, stir in the coconut milk, and lemon juice. Let it stand for 5 minutes.

Add into half of the flour mixture the eggs and milk and mix until well combined.

Fold in the berries.

Pour the mixture into the prepared pan and sprinkle on top the reserved crumb topping.

Bake for 50 minutes.

Allow to cool before slicing.

Nutrition: Calories 171, Total Fat 12.7g, Saturated Fat 8.2g, Total Carbs 13.6g, Net Carbs 13g, Protein 1.9g, Sugar: 10.1g, Fiber: 0.6g, Sodium: 107mg, Potassium: 70mg

Chocolate Chunks Cookies

Preparation Time: 8 hours, Cooking Time: 15 minutes

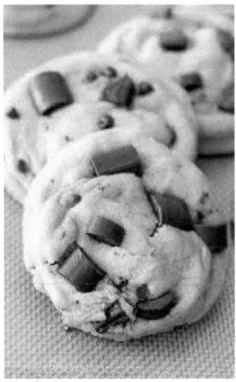

Servings: 14

Ingredients:

2 1/3 cup gluten-free flour

1 teaspoon baking soda

1 cup unsalted butter, room temperature

1 cup light brown sugar

2 teaspoons vanilla extract

2 large eggs

12 oz dark chocolates, chopped

1 1/3 cups toasted pecan halves, chopped

1 teaspoon salt

Direction:

In a bowl, mix together the flour, baking soda, and salt. Sift the flour mixture to aerate. Set aside.

Place the butter in a bowl and add in the sugar and vanilla extract. Beat for 3 minutes until the mixture lightens. Add in the eggs one at a time.

Beat in the dry mixture until only a few streaks of flour remain.

Stir in the dark chocolates and pecans until well combined. Cover the bowl and chill for at least 4 hours.

Preheat the oven to 3750F. Line a baking sheet with parchment paper. Position the rack in the upper thirds of the oven.

Form small balls from the dough and place on the baking sheet.

Bake for 15 minutes or until lightly brown.

Nutrition: Calories 378, Total Fat 26.7g, Saturated Fat 12.3g, Total Carbs 32.2g, Net Carbs 28.5g, Protein 4.1g, Sugar: 21.7g, Fiber: 3.7g, Sodium: 47mg, Potassium: 262mg

Peanut Butter Oatmeal Chocolate Chip Cookies

Preparation Time: 20 minutes, Cook time:15 minutes

Servings: 14

Ingredients:

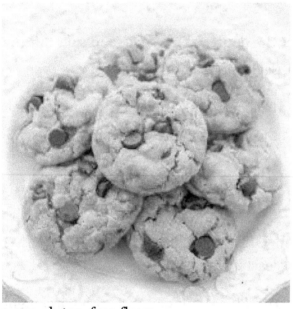

1 cup gluten-free flour

½ teaspoon xanthan gum

1 teaspoon baking soda

8 tablespoons unsalted butter, cold and cubed

½ cup natural creamy peanut butter

2/3 cup sugar

1 teaspoon pure vanilla extract

1 large egg

¾ cup gluten-free quick oats

1 cup semi-sweet mini chocolate chips

¼ teaspoon salt

Direction:

Preheat the oven to 3500F. Line a baking sheet with parchment paper.

In a small bowl, mix together the gluten-free flour, xanthan gum, baking soda, and salt.

In another bowl, cream the butter and add in the peanut butter, sugar, and vanilla extract. Beat in the eggs and continue to beat until well-combined.

Gradually add the dry ingredients and mix until everything is incorporated.

Stir in the oats, chocolate chip cookies. Scoop the cookie dough and place on the cookie sheet.

Bake for 12 minutes.

Remove from the cookie sheet on the cooling rack before serving.

Nutrition: Calories 199, Total Fat 10.3g, Saturated Fat 3.9g, Total Carbs 25.5g, Net Carbs 23.6, Protein 4.2g, Sugar: 15.8g, Fiber: 1.9g, Sodium: 65mg, Potassium: 161mg

Baked Peanut Butter Protein Bars

Preparation Time: 20 minutes

Cooking Time: 0 minutes

Servings: 12

Ingredients:

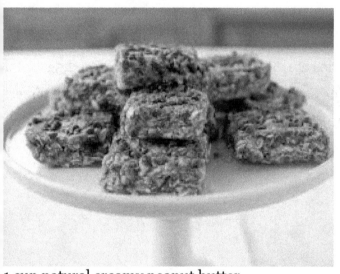

1 cup natural creamy peanut butter

¾ cup maple syrup

1 teaspoon vanilla bean paste

1 ½ cups gluten-free rolled oats

1 cup protein powder

Direction:

Line a baking pan with parchment paper.

In a microwave-safe bowl, heat the peanut butter and maple syrup for 30 seconds. Stir then add in the vanilla bean paste then heat again for 30 seconds.

Stir in oats and protein powder.

Spread into the prepared pan and press using the back of the spoon.

Refrigerate for an hour and cut into 12 bars.

Nutrition: Calories 271, Total Fat 14.9g, Saturated Fat 2.5g, Total Carbs 27.6g, Net Carbs 23.4g, Protein 14g, Sugar: 13.7g, Fiber: 4.2g, Sodium: 128mg, Potassium: 442mg

Gluten-Free Lemon Cookies

Preparation Time: 20 minutes

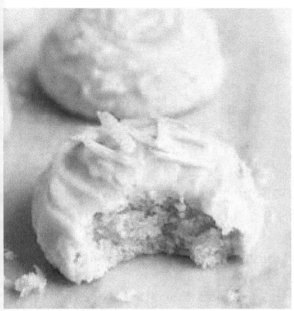

Cooking Time: 15 minutes

Servings: 20

Ingredients:

¼ cup coconut milk

¼ cup fresh lemon juice

½ cup butter

1 egg

1 teaspoon vanilla extract

Zest of one lemon

1 teaspoon baking soda

1 teaspoon baking powder

2 ½ cups gluten-free flour

½ cup fresh lemon juice

2 cups powdered sugar

1 cup sugar

Direction:

Preheat the oven to 3500F and grease a baking sheet with butter. Set aside.

Combine the milk and lemon juice in a bowl. Set aside.

Cream the butter and sugar using an electric mixer. Add in the egg and vanilla extract.

Add in the milk mixture to the butter mixture and fold. Set aside.

In another bowl, combine the lemon zest, baking powder, and flour.

Add the dry ingredients to the wet ingredients then fold.

Scoop cookie dough and place on the baking sheet. Press the dough using your fingers.

Bake for 15 minutes.

Allow the cookies to cool on a cooling rack.

Meanwhile, prepare the frosting by mixing the lemon juice and sugar.

Brush the top of the cookies with the frosting.

Nutrition: Calories 110, Total Fat 5.9g, Saturated Fat 3.7g, Total Carbs 14.1g, Net Carbs 13.9g, Protein 0.9g, Sugar:10.3 g, Fiber: 0.2g, Sodium: 65mg, Potassium: 40mg

Granola Bars

Preparation Time: 15 minutes

Cooking Time: 15 minutes

Servings: 12

Ingredients:

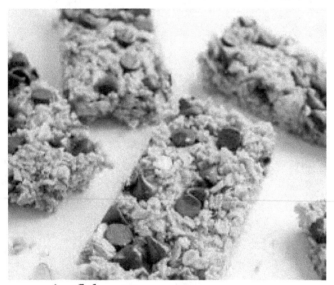

1 cup rice flake

1 cup millet flakes

½ cup dried cranberries

½ cup pumpkin seeds

¼ cup sunflower seeds

½ cup peanut butter

2 teaspoons malt syrup

1 teaspoon cinnamon powder

Coconut oil for greasing

Direction:

Preheat the oven to 3550F and grease a small baking tray.

In a bowl, mix together the rice flakes, millet, cranberries, pumpkin seeds, and peanut butter.

In a blender, mix together the peanut butter, and malt syrup. Add in the cinnamon powder.

Pour into the granola mixture and mix well.

Press into the baking tray and bake for 15 minutes.

Allow to harden before cutting into bars.

Nutrition: Calories 180, Total Fat 8.6g, Saturated Fat 1.4g, Total Carbs 23.4g, Net Carbs 19g, Protein 6.1g, Sugar: 4.4g, Fiber: 4.4g, Sodium: 175mg, Potassium: 270mg

Cocoa Lemon Bites

Preparation Time: 5 minutes

Cooking Time: 10 minutes

Servings: 10

Ingredients:

1 cup pecans

3 Tbsp. maple syrup

2 ½ tsp lemon juice

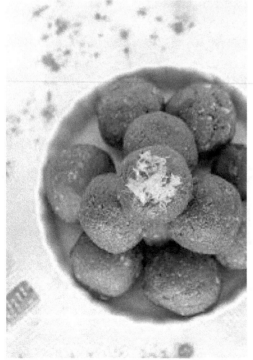

1 tsp lemon zest

2 tsp cinnamon

2 Tbsp. cocoa powder

½ tsp vanilla

¼ tsp salt

Direction:

Mix the Ingredients and blend using a food processor.

Shape into balls

Serve immediately

Nutrition: Calories: 192, Saturated Fat: 2.9g, Cholesterol: 0mg, Sodium: 22mg, Total Carbohydrates: 35g, Dietary Fiber: 4.9g, Potassium: 46mg, Iron: 1mg, Calcium: 21mg, Protein: 2.9g, Total sugars: 25.2g

Fudge Brownies

Preparation Time: 10 minutes

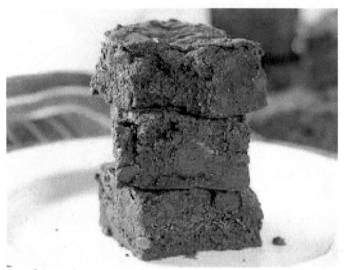

Cooking time: 30 minutes

Servings: 16

Ingredients:

2 large eggs

2/3 cup all-purpose flour, gluten-free

1 tsp vanilla

1 cup granulated sugar

½ cup unsweetened cocoa powder

½ cup butter

½ tsp salt

Direction:

Preheat the oven to 350 0 F.

Spray a baking pan with cooking spray and set aside.

Melt butter in a saucepan over low heat.

Remove saucepan from heat. Add cocoa powder and stir until smooth.

Beat in eggs, vanilla, and sugar.

Add flour and salt and stir until well combined.

Pour batter in the prepared baking pan and spread evenly.

Bake in preheated oven for 25-30 minutes.

Remove from oven and let it cool completely.

Slice and serve.

Nutrition: Calories: 133, Total Fat: 6.8g, Saturated Fat: 4.1g, Protein: 1.9g, Carbs: 18g, Fiber: 1g, Sugar: 12.6g

Chocolate Protein Balls

Preparation Time: 2 hours 10 minutes

Servings: 10

Ingredients:

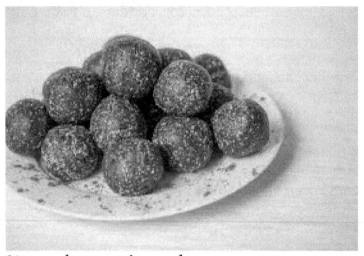

¾ cup whey protein powder

2 Tbsp. fresh orange juice

1 Tbsp. chia seeds

1 Tbsp. cocoa powder

2 Tbsp. maple syrup

¼ cup peanut butter

½ tsp orange zest

Direction:

Add all Ingredients into the bowl and mix until well combined.

Make ten small balls from mixture and place on a plate.

Place in refrigerator for 2 hours.

Serve and enjoy.

Nutrition: Calories: 70, Total Fat: 4g, Saturated Fat: 0.9g, Protein: 4.1g, Carbs: 5.4g, Fiber: 0.6g, Sugar: 3.5g

Garlic-Infused Croutons

Cooking Time: 15 minutes

Servings: 4

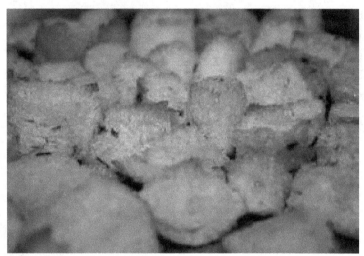

Ingredients:

8 slices stale wheat bread, cubed

4 teaspoons garlic-infused oil

3 tablespoons butter

½ teaspoon oregano, dried

Rock salt

Direction:

Set the oven to 170 degrees Celsius.

Place the garlic-infused oil and butter in a bowl. Microwave on high while covered for 20 seconds.

Coat the bread cubes with the butter mixture. Season with salt and oregano.

Arrange the bread cubes in a single layer on a roasting tray. Bake for 15 minutes. Turn the bread once during the cook.

Nutrition: 285 calories, 35.3 mg calcium, 14.9 g fat, 2.5 mg iron, 2.2 g saturates, 2.8 g sugars, 0.5 g salt, 6.5 g protein, 1.4 g fiber and 31.5 g carbohydrates.

Frozen Banana Bites

Cooking Time: 6 hours

Servings: 3

Ingredients:

3 medium firm bananas, sliced

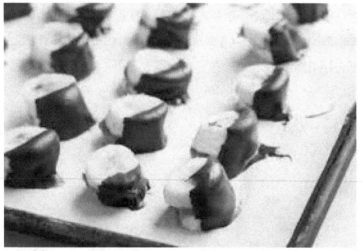

3 tablespoons sunflower seeds, toasted and chopped

100 g dark chocolate, melted

4 tablespoons peanut butter

3 tablespoons sprinkles

4 tablespoons low FODMAP muesli

2 tablespoons coconut, dried and shredded

Direction:

Coat half of each banana slices with chocolate and sprinkle topping of choice on top.

Arrange the banana slices in a square pan lined with baking paper. Freeze for 5 hours.

Nutrition: 604 calories, 50 mg calcium, 38 g fat, 5.3 mg iron, 17.4 g saturates, 8.8 g fiber, 11 g protein, 31.8 g sugars and 61.2 g carbohydrates.

Salted Caramel Pumpkin Seeds

Cooking Time: 25 minutes

Servings: 16

Ingredients:

284 g pumpkin seeds

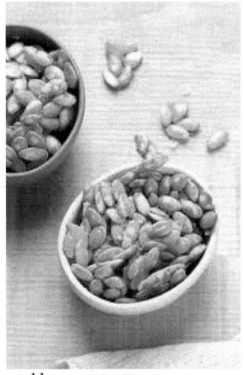

2 tablespoons water

½ teaspoon ginger, ground

3 ½ teaspoons white sugar

1/8 teaspoon nutmeg, ground

¼ teaspoon cinnamon, ground

1 ½ tablespoons butter

½ teaspoon rock salt

1 ½ tablespoon brown sugar

Direction:

Set the oven to 150 degrees Celsius.

Combine pumpkin seeds, water, 2 ½ teaspoons white sugar, cinnamon, nutmeg and ginger together in a large bowl.

Use baking paper to line a roasting tray and drizzle with oil. Distribute the pumpkin seeds evenly on the tray.

Bake in the oven for 25 minutes.

Over medium flame, heat the butter in a large saucepan until melted. Add remaining ingredients and mix well. Cook for 2 minutes.

Reduce heat to low. Transfer the seeds to the saucepan and coat completely with sauce.

Return the seeds to the roasting tray to cool.

Nutrition: 130 calories, 9.7 mg calcium, 9.8 g fat, 1.6 mg iron, 1.7 g saturates, 5.7 g sugars, 0.1 g salt, 5.4 g protein, 1.1 g fiber and 7.4 g carbohydrates.

Ginger Cookies

Cooking Time: 30 minutes

Servings: 26

Ingredients:

190 g butter

1 teaspoon guar gum

208 g white sugar

¼ teaspoon s alt

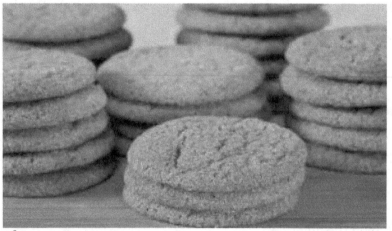

1 large egg

½ teaspoon cloves, ground

60 g golden syrup

¾ teaspoon cinnamon, ground

350 g plain flour, gluten-free

1 teaspoon baking soda

2 teaspoon ginger, ground

Direction:

Set the oven to 180 degrees Celsius.

Mix sugar and butter together until fluffy. Add golden egg and syrup. Whisk ingredients until well combined.

Place flour, guar gum, ginger, salt, cinnamon, cloves and baking soda in a separate bowl. Stir well.

Combine the two mixtures and mix well.

Using a spoon, place equal amounts of the cookie mixture in two cookie trays lined with baking paper. Space the cookies evenly.

Press each cookie slightly to flatten them. Sprinkle sugar on top.

Cook in the oven for 12 minutes. Set aside to cool.

Nutrition: 146 calories, 20.1 mg calcium, 6.1 g fat, 0.3 mg iron, 0.9 g saturates, 10.2 g sugars, 0.1-gram salt, 1.2 g protein, 0.2 g fiber and 21.2 g carbohydrates.

Orange Delight Biscuits

Cooking Time: 25 minutes

Servings: 24

Ingredients:

½ teaspoon baking soda

1 teaspoon vanilla extract

½ teaspoon salt

3 ½ table spoons fresh orange juice

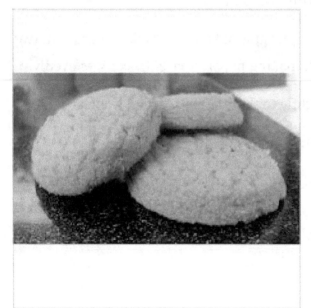

280 g plain flour, gluten-free

1 large egg

2 ½ teaspoons orange zest, grated

210 g white sugar

115 g butter

130 g powdered sugar

Direction:

Set the oven to 180 degrees Celsius.

Place salt, 1 teaspoon orange zest, baking soda and flour in a large bowl. Mix well.

Whisk together sugar and butter in a separate bowl until fluffy. Add 2 tablespoons orange juice, vanilla extract and egg. Stir well.

Combine the two mixtures together. Scoop dough balls in cookie trays lined with baking paper. Press each ball lightly to flatten.

Cook in the oven for 10 minutes. Rotate the trays and bake for another 10 minutes. Set aside to cool.

Mix remaining ingredients together to create orange icing. Apply mixture on top of each biscuit.

Nutrition: 172 calories, 71.8 mg calcium, 4.2 g fat, 0.5 mg iron, 0.7 g saturates, 14.6 g sugars, 0.1-gram salt, 1.6 g protein, 3.6 g fiber and 32.5 g carbohydrates.

Lemon Cake

Cooking Time: 25 minutes

Servings: 12

Ingredients:

105 g self-rising flour, gluten-free

3 tablespoons lemon zest

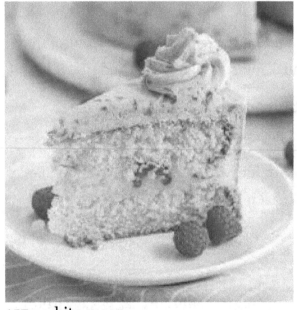

157 g white sugar

3 ½ tablespoons lemon juice

¼ teaspoon salt

2 large eggs

100 g butter, softened

Direction:

Set the oven to 180 degrees Celsius.

Place flour, sugar, butter and salt in a bowl and mix until doughy.

Stir together the eggs, lemon juice and zest in a separate bowl.

Combine the two mixtures together and whisk until smooth.

Transfer mixture into a baking pan greased with oil. Cook in the oven for 25 minutes. Set aside to cool.

To create the icing, mix remaining lemon juice and powdered sugar together.

Spread icing on top of the cake after it cooled. Distribute lemon zest on top. Cut the cake once icing has set.

Nutrition: 204 calories, 19.5 mg calcium, 7.7 g fat, 0.4 mg iron, 1.3 g saturates, 24.2 g sugars, 0.1-gram salt, 1.9 g protein, 0.2 g fiber and 31.9 g carbohydrates.

Blueberry Crumble

Cooking Time: 30 minutes

Servings: 12

Ingredients:

208 g white sugar

1 large egg

420 g self-rising flour, gluten-free

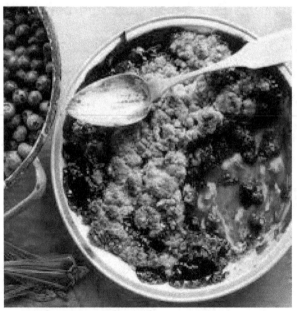

250 g butter, softened

¼ teaspoon salt

1 teaspoon guar gum

½ teaspoon cinnamon, ground

3 teaspoons corn starch

445 g fresh blueberries

Direction:

Set the oven to 180 degrees Celsius.

Mix 156 g sugar, salt, 420 g flour and cinnamon together. Add guar gum and mix well.

Whisk the eggs slightly with butter. Pour resulting mixture into the dry ingredients. Stir until well combined.

Press half of the mixture into a lightly greased baking pan until a smooth layer is formed.

Spread the blueberries on top of the dough evenly.

Combine corn starch and remaining sugar together. Sprinkle mixture on top of blueberries.

Crumble remaining dough mixture using your fingers. Spread crumbs on top of the blueberry mixture.

Cook in the oven for 30 minutes. Allow to cool before slicing.

Nutrition: 307 calories, 40.8 mg calcium, 13.9 g fat, 0.7 milligram iron, 2.1 g saturates, 17.7 g sugars, 0.2-gram salt, 2.6 g protein, 1-gram fiber and 42.1 g carbohydrates.

Crispy Roasted Potatoes

Cooking Time: 1 hour

Servings: 4

Ingredients:

800 g potatoes, sliced

1/8 teaspoon chili flakes, dried

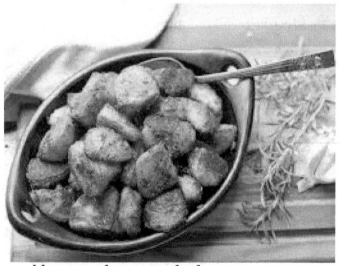

4 tablespoons butter, melted

¼ teaspoon sea salt

1 ½ teaspoon fresh thyme

Salt and pepper

Direction:

Set the oven to 190 degrees Celsius.

Grease an oven-proof fry pan using 1 tablespoon butter.

Arrange potato slices in an upright position. Drizzle with remaining butter. Distribute thyme and chili flakes on top. Season to taste.

Cook in the oven for an hour then set aside to cool for 10 minutes.

Nutrition: 257 calories, 26.1 mg calcium, 11.4 g fat, 1.7 mg iron, 1.7 g saturates, 1.6 g sugars, 0.3-gram salt, 4.2 g protein, 4.3 g fiber and 35.3 g carbohydrates.

Chocolate Zucchini Cake

Cooking Time: 50 minutes

Servings: 16

Ingredients:

500 g zucchini, shredded

1 teaspoon baking powder

250 milliliters canola oil

280 g plain flour, gluten-free

200 g brown sugar

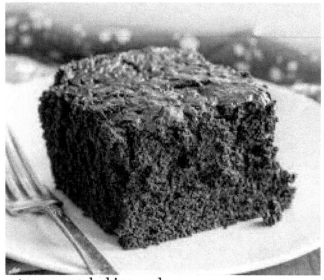

2 teaspoons baking soda

2 teaspoons chia seeds

½ teaspoon salt

1 teaspoon cinnamon, ground

3 large eggs

65 g cocoa powder

100 g butter, soft

20 g dark chocolate, grated

195 g powdered sugar

Boiling water

Direction:

Set the oven to 175 degrees Celsius.

Soak chia seeds in 4 teaspoons boiling water to soften.

Whisk oil, eggs, brown sugar, salt, chia seed mixture, cinnamon and cocoa powder together in a large bowl.

Dissolve baking soda in 1 tablespoon of warm water. Add to the egg mixture and stir well.

Place baking powder and flour in a large bowl and mix well.

Combine the two mixtures together in a food processor. Add zucchini and stir until well combined.

Pour batter into a greased baking tin. Bake for 50 minutes then remove from oven to cool.

Put remaining ingredients together in a bowl. Add boiling water and mix until desired consistency is reached.

Coat the cake evenly with icing.

Nutrition: 387 calories, 70.3 mg calcium, 23.3 g fat, 1.6 mg iron, 3 g saturates, 25.8 g sugars, 0.3 g salt, 4.1 g protein, 2.4 g fiber and 43.4 g carbohydrates.

Chocolate Brownie Cupcakes with Vanilla Icing

Cooking Time: 20 minutes

Servings: 12

Ingredients:

225 g butter

½ teaspoon salt

100 g dark chocolate, chopped

¼ teaspoon baking soda

2 large eggs

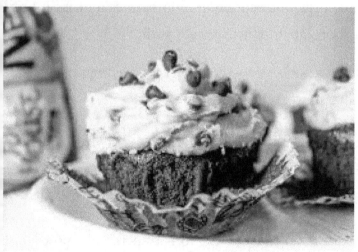

¾ teaspoon baking powder

63 milliliters almond milk

150 g brown sugar

1 ½ teaspoon vanilla extract

3 tablespoons cocoa powder

140 g plain flour, gluten-free

195 g powdered sugar

Red food coloring

Direction:

Set the oven to 170 degrees Celsius.

Microwave 125 g butter and chocolate on high for 15 seconds then stir. Do it repeatedly until chocolate is melted.

Whisk together eggs, 1 teaspoon vanilla extract and milk until smooth. Add chocolate mixture and stir well.

Place flour, baking soda, cocoa powder, salt, baking powder and brown sugar in a bowl and mix well.

Combine the two mixtures together. Pour the batter into the muffin tray lined with paper cups.

Bake for 15 minutes. Once done, set aside to cool.

Slightly heat the remaining butter to soften it. Add powdered sugar, vanilla extract and 2 drops of food coloring. Stir until smooth.

Pipe icing on top of each cupcake.

Nutrition: 365 calories, 60.6 mg calcium, 19.9 g fat, 1.8 mg iron, 4.7 g saturates, 30.8 g sugars, 0.3 g salt, 3.2 g protein, 1.7 g fiber and 43.9 g carbohydrates.

Rhubarb and Strawberry Crumble

Cooking Time: 35 minutes

Servings: 3

Ingredients:

130 g fresh rhubarb, peeled and sliced

4 tablespoons butter, softened

2 tablespoons water

2 tablespoons pumpkin seeds

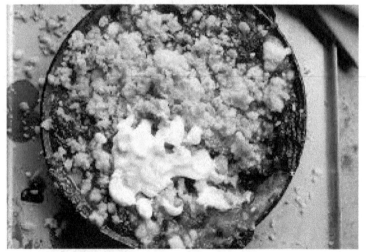

140 g frozen strawberries, quartered

3 tablespoons dried coconut, shredded

1 ½ teaspoon white sugar

35 g plain flour, gluten-free

1 tablespoon corn starch

50 g brown sugar

50 g gluten-free cornflakes, crushed

Direction:

Set the oven to 200 degrees Celsius.

Place water, 1 tablespoon sugar and rhubarb in a baking tray. Roast for 10 minutes.

Once tender, remove from oven and reduce heat to 180 degrees Celsius.

Combine cornflakes, pumpkin seeds, brown sugar, coconut and flour together in a small bowl. Add butter and mix until crumbly.

Put rhubarb, strawberries, corn starch and sugar in an oven dish. Distribute crumble mixture evenly on top.

Bake for 20 minutes.

Nutrition: 425 calories, 79.7 mg calcium, 22.2 g fat, 3.1 mg iron, 5.7 g saturates, 22.6 g sugars, 0.3 g salt, 5.7 g protein, 3.6 g fiber and 52.2 g carbohydrates.

Vanilla Lemon Cookies

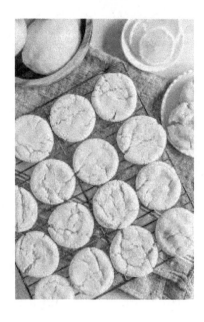

Cooking Time: 1 hour

Servings: 25

Ingredients:

200 g butter, softened

2 tablespoons almond milk

150 g white sugar

1 teaspoon guar gum

2 egg yolks

400 g plain flour, gluten-free

1 tablespoon lemon zest

1 teaspoon vanilla extract

200 g dark chocolate

3 tablespoons sprinkles

Direction:

Set the oven to 180 degrees Celsius.

Mix sugar and butter together until fluffy. Whisk in egg yolks and vanilla extract.

Add flour, milk and lemon zest. Mix well.

Lightly knead the dough. Flatten the mixture to ¼-inch thickness using a rolling pin. Cut into desired shapes.

Put the cookies in a square pan lined with baking paper. Bake for 15 minutes then remove from the oven to cool.

Mix 6 teaspoons sugar and dark chocolate together in a double broiler until melted. Dip each cookie in the chocolate mixture and top with sprinkles.

Nutrition: 209 calories, 29.9 mg calcium, 10.7 g fat, 1.3 mg iron, 3.5 g saturates, 10.4 g sugars, 0.1-gram salt, 1.9 g protein, 1-gram fiber and 25.5 g carbohydrates.

Strawberry Popsicle

Cooking Time: 4 hours

Servings: 3

Ingredients:

140 g strawberries, chopped

2 teaspoons pure maple syrup

125 milliliters almond milk

1 teaspoon vanilla extract

63 milliliters coconut yogurt

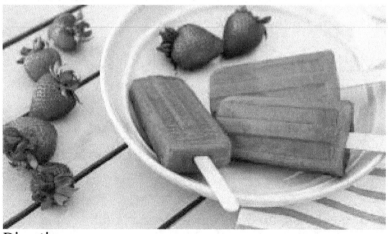

Direction:

Place all of the ingredients in a food processor. Blend until smooth.

Pour mixture into popsicle holders. Freeze for 4 hours.

Nutrition: 66 calories, 82.5 mg calcium, 0.9 g fat, 0.4 mg iron, 0.2 g saturates, 1.4 g fiber, 1.1 g protein, 8.1 g sugars and 13.3 g carbohydrates.

Macadamia nuts Cheesecake with Blueberries

Makes a small cake (18 cm), 12 portions for the base

120 gr of pecans

50 gr of almond flour

20 gr of extra-virgin coconut oil (melted)

20 gr of maple syrup

For the middle layer

220 gr of macadamia nuts

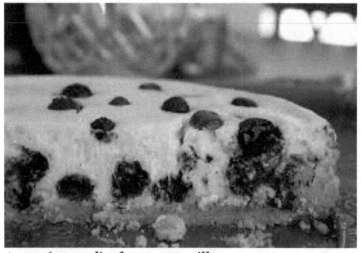

A can (350 ml) of coconut milk

60 ml of lemon (or lime) juice

4 tablespoons of maple syrup

1/2 teaspoon vanilla powder

For the top layer

280 gr of blueberries

Half a glass of water

1 tablespoon of maple syrup (optional)

A splash of lemon juice

Vanilla powder, to taste

Direction:

The night before, put the macadamia nuts in a bowl, and cover them with warm water. Leave them to soak overnight (or at least for 6-8 hours). Also place the coconut milk tin in the refrigerator, so that the fatty part separates from the more liquid part.

In a bowl, combine the pecan flour along with the almond flour, the extra virgin coconut oil (melted) and the maple syrup. Mix well and put the mixture into the cake pan, pressing with the back of a spoon to make base for the cake evenly spread. Put the base in the refrigerator to set.

Meanwhile prepare the middle layer: in a large blender put the macadamia nuts previously soaked and drained well. Then open the coconut milk can and remove the solid part only, which should be now on the surface (you can use the liquid part to make other recipes, such as smoothies). Combine the coconut cream with the macadamia nuts.

Then add the other ingredients: lemon juice, vanilla powder and maple syrup.

Blend everything until the mixture reaches a creamy consistency. Pour the mixture over the base; and put everything in the freezer for at least an hour to set.

Meanwhile prepare the top layer: in a saucepan pour the well washed blueberries, add half cup of water, lemon juice, vanilla and maple syrup. Cook over low heat until the blueberry compote thickens (about 40 minutes). Let it cool completely and then pour on the cake.

Place the cake in the freezer. I suggest you remove it from the freezer half an hour before serving.

Nutrition: 209 calories, 29.9 mg calcium, 10.7 g fat, 1.3 mg iron, 3.5 g saturates, 10.4 g sugars, 0.1-gram salt, 1.9 g protein, 1-gram fiber and 25.5 g carbohydrates.

Pumpkin and Chocolate Cake

Ingredients (10-12 serves)

300 gr pumpkin, steamed and puréed

130 gr allowed flour / flour mix*

4 eggs

100 gr maple syrup

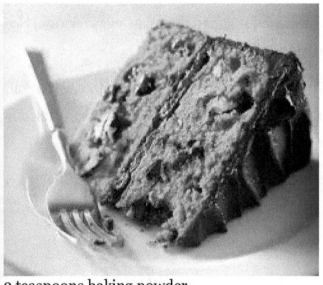

2 teaspoons baking powder

4 teaspoons cocoa powder

130 gr dark chocolate (cocoa min. 70%)

75 gr extra-virgin coconut oil

A bit of salt and a bit of vanilla powder

Direction:

Break the eggs and separate the egg whites from the yolks

Beat the egg whites until stiff, then put them in the refrigerator.

Melt the chocolate pieces together with the coconut oil in hot water. Let it cool for 5 minutes.

In a medium-sized bowl, combine and mix flour, cocoa, vanilla powder, yeast and salt.

With another bowl, mix well steamed pumpkin, egg yolks and rice syrup using an electric mixer.

To this mixture, first add the melted chocolate with coconut oil, then the dry ingredients and finally the egg whites, stirring slowly from the bottom to the top.

Pour all the mixture into a 22 cm diameter baking pan with parchment paper.

Bake for 40/45 minutes at 180/190°C.

Notes * You can make your own low FODMAP flour mix using, for instance, 50 gr rice flour, 25 gr cornstarch, 25 gr potato starch, 30 gr oatmeal. Or 65 gr rice flour and 65 gr buckwheat. Depending on the consistency you want to get.

Nutrition: 123 calories, 29 mg calcium, 10.7 g fat, 1 mg iron, 5 g saturates, 14 g sugars, 0.1-gram salt, 1.9 g protein, 1-gram fiber and 25 g carbohydrates.

Walnuts and Banana Brownie

Ingredients (8/10 portions)

50 g rice flour

30 g almond meal

2 teaspoons of baking powder

150 g extra-virgin coconut oil

130 g Demerara sugar

130 g dark chocolate, chopped (min 70%)

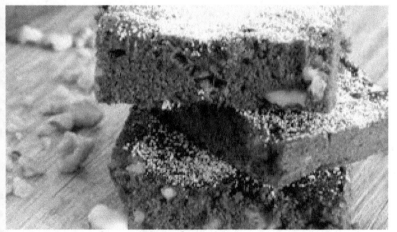

4 teaspoons of cocoa powder

1 banana, mashed

2 large eggs

40 g walnuts (or Brazil nuts), chopped

Direction:

Melt the extra-virgin coconut oil with the chocolate and let it cool.

In a bowl mix flour, almond meal, baking powder and cocoa.

In another bowl beat eggs, sugar and mashed banana with an electric mixer.

Add the chocolate and coconut oil mixture and mix.

Add the dry ingredients (flour, almond meal, baking powder and cocoa) and mix well.

Finally add chopped walnuts.

Put your mixture in a baking dish (22 cm diameter) and cook for 40/45 minutes at 180/190° C.

Nutrition: 229 calories, 29.9 mg calcium, 10.7 g fat, 1.3 mg iron, 7 g saturates, 10.4 g sugars, 0.1-gram salt, 1.9 g protein, 1-gram fiber and 35 g carbohydrates.

Pumpkin Pie

Preparation time: 15 minutes

Cooking time: 60 minutes

Serves 8

Ingredients:

150 g granulated sugar

1 tsp g round cinnamon

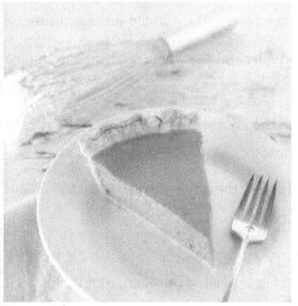

½ tsp salt

½ tsp ground ginger

¼ tsp ground cloves

2 eggs

230 g can of pure pumpkin

350 ml vanilla creamer

1 unbaked 9-inch FODMAP Free pie crust – either bought or made

Direction:

Preheat oven to 425° F

Put the sugar, cinnamon, ginger, salt and cloves in a bowl and mix well

Beat the eggs in a separate bowl and stir in the sugar mixture

Stir the creamer in gradually and the whole mixture into the pie shell

Bake for 15 minutes and then reduce the heat to 350° F and bake for a further 40-50 minutes

Cool for 2 hours on a wire rack the serve with low FODMAP cream or refrigerate

Nutrition: 231 calories, 19 mg calcium, 10.7 g fat, 1.3 mg iron, 5 g saturates, 14 g sugars, 0.1-gram salt, 9 g protein, 1-gram fiber and 25 g carbohydrates.

Almond Cake

Preparation time: 35 minutes Cooking time: 75 minutes Serves 10

Ingredients

250 g softened dairy free butter

75 g castor sugar

4 eggs

240 g finely ground almonds

40 g rice flour

Low FODMAP cream to serve

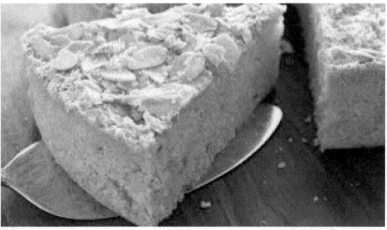

Direction:

Preheat the oven to 320° F

Grease a pan, 6 cm deep and 22 cm round and then line it with baking paper

Beat the butter and the sugar using a hand mixer, until light and fluffy

Add the eggs one at a time, beating after each one

Stir the finely chopped almonds and flour into the mix

Spread over the pan and bake for 75 minutes or until cooked through

Leave to cool in the pan for 10 minutes, then turn out onto a wire rack and cool for a further 10 minutes

Serves with the cream and fresh fruit of your choice

Nutrition: 209 calories, 29.9 mg calcium, 10.7 g fat, 1.3 mg iron, 3.5 g saturates, 10.4 g sugars, 0.1-gram salt, 1.9 g protein, 1-gram fiber and 25.5 g carbohydrates.

Instant Banana Pudding

Preparation time: 10 minutes

Cooking time: 60 minutes

Serves 12

Ingredients:

140 g box of Jell-O vanilla instant pudding

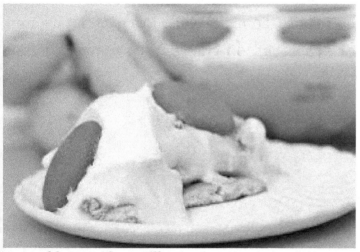

600 ml lactose free milk

150 g pack of gluten free cookies

3 whole bananas, peeled

Direction:

Whisk the pudding mix and milk together for 2 minutes until the pudding begins to thicken

Place in the refrigerator to continue thickening

Slice the bananas and divide into two piles

Break up the cookies and spread half of them over the base of an 8 x 8 pan

Place half of the bananas over the top and follow with half of the pudding mix

Repeat with the rest of the ingredients

Nutrition: 200 calories, 20 mg calcium, 10.7 g fat, 1.3 mg iron, 3.5 g saturates, 14 g sugars, 0.1-gram salt, 1.9 g protein, 1-gram fiber and 15 g carbohydrates.

Chocolate-Orange-Raspberry Cupcakes

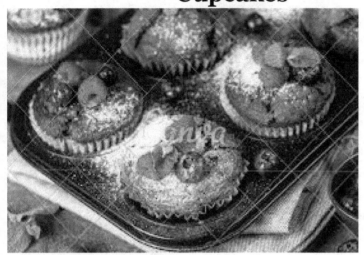

Preparation time: 15 minutes

Cooking time: 30 minutes

Serves 24

Ingredients:

360 ml almond milk

120 ml unsweetened orange juice

1 tsp rice vinegar

450 g Turbinado sugar

160 ml vegetable oil

2 eggs

200 g oat flour

½ tsp xanthan gum

35 g cocoa powder

1 tsp baking soda

1 tsp baking powder

½ tsp salt

2 tsp orange zest

2 tbsp. organic raspberry preserves

1 tsp vanilla

Direction:

Preheat oven to 350° F

Line a cupcake tin with molds

Mix the vinegar, milk and orange juice together and leave to curdle for 5 minutes

Mic the flour, xanthan gum, baking powder, baking soda, cocoa and salt together

Beat the eggs in a separate bowl with the oil, sugar and orange zest

Mix the flour mix and the milk into the egg mix, alternating each one to ensure even mixing and beat until the mixture is smooth and well combined

Spoon into the molds and bake for 30 minutes

Leave to cool while you make the frosting

Nutrition: 209 calories, 29.9 mg calcium, 10.7 g fat, 1.3 mg iron, 3.5 g saturates, 10.4 g sugars, 0.1-gram salt, 1.9 g protein, 1-gram fiber and 25.5 g carbohydrates.

Chocolate-Orange-Raspberry Frosting

Ingredients:

770 g sifted powdered sugar

2 tbsp. unsweetened cocoa powder

½ tsp salt

60 ml almond milk

675 g dairy-free butter

1 tsp vanilla extract

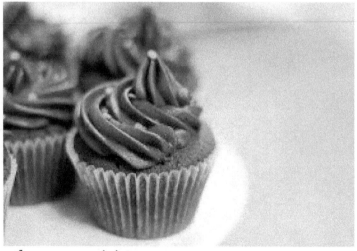

1 tbsp. orange juice

2 tsp organic raspberry preserves

Orange zest - for flavor and/or garnish

Direction:

Mix the sugar with the salt and cocoa powder

Using an electric mixer, mix the milk, orange juice and raspberry jelly together for about 5 minutes or until smooth

Add the vanilla and butter and beat for a further 10 minutes

Frost the cupcakes and serve

Nutrition: 199 calories, 29.9 mg calcium, 10.7 g fat, 1.3 mg iron, 3.5 g saturates, 10.4 g sugars, 0.1-gram salt, 1.9 g protein, 1-gram fiber and 25.5 g carbohydrates.

Graham Crackers

Preparation time: 140 minutes

Cooking time: 20 minutes

Makes 10 crackers

Ingredients:

325 g all-purpose flour, gluten free, sifted

2 extra tbsp. gluten free all-purpose flour

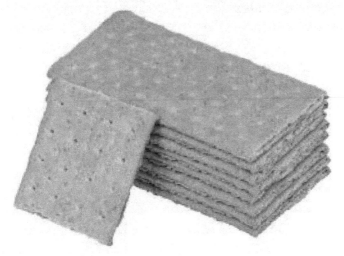

2 ½ tsp xanthan gum

170 g dark brown sugar

1 tsp baking soda

¾ tsp coarse sea salt

7 tbsp. dairy free butter – cut into cubes of 1" and freeze in advance

90 g molasses

5 tablespoons lactose free whole milk

2 tbsp. clear vanilla extract

3 tbsp. granulated sugar

1 tsp ground cinnamon

Direction:

Mix the flour together with the xanthan gum, brown sugar, baking soda, and salt in a food processor using a steel blade or in and electric mixer using the paddle

Either pule or lave on a low setting to thoroughly mix

Ass in the frozen cubes of butter and pulse until the mixture looks like coarse meal

Whisk the vanilla, molasses and milk together in a separate bowl

Add the liquid into the dry mixture and pulse until the mixture is a soft and sticky dough that only just comes together

Dust a large piece of plastic wrap with flour (gluten free) and turn the dough out onto it

Pat and shape into a 1" thick rectangle, wrap it up and chill in the refrigerator until firm, around 2 hours

Mix the granulated sugar and the cinnamon together and leave to one side

When the dough is chilled divide it in half and put half back in the refrigerator

Sprinkle flour evenly on the work surface and roll out the dough into a long rectangle, around 1/8" thick. It will be sticky so use more flour as and when you need it but make sure it is gluten free

Cut the dough up into rectangles that are 4 ½" by 4" approximately

Place them onto a baking sheet lined with baking paper and sprinkle the sugar and cinnamon mix over the top ad place in the refrigerator for about 30-45 minutes or until firm (alternatively, pop the tray in the freezer for 15-20 minutes)

Repeat the process with the other half of the dough and then, with any scraps that are left over

While the crackers are chilling, preheat the oven to 350° F

Bake the crackers for 15-25 minutes or until they have browned and are a little firm to the touch. Make sure you rotate the baking trays halfway through cooking to make sure they are evenly baked